MINDFULNESS-BASED THERAPY FOR MANAGING FATIGUE

Mindfulness-Based Therapy *for* Managing Fatigue

Supporting People with ME/CFS, Fibromyalgia and Long Covid

Fiona McKechnie

Forewords by Professor Rebecca Crane and Dh Taravajra

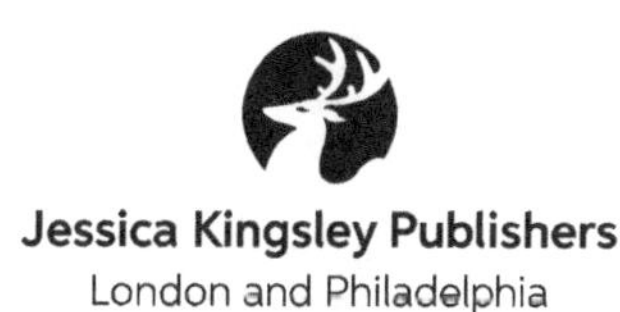

Jessica Kingsley Publishers
London and Philadelphia

First published in Great Britain in 2024 by Jessica Kingsley Publishers
An imprint of John Murray Press

2

A CIP catalogue record for this title is available from the
British Library and the Library of Congress

ISBN 978 1 83997 345 1
eISBN 978 1 83997 346 8

Printed and bound by CPI Group (UK) Ltd, Croydon, CR0 4YY

Jessica Kingsley Publishers' policy is to use papers that are natural, renewable and recyclable products and made from wood grown in sustainable forests. The logging and manufacturing processes are expected to conform to the environmental regulations of the country of origin.

Jessica Kingsley Publishers
Carmelite House
50 Victoria Embankment
London EC4Y 0DZ

www.jkp.com

John Murray Press
Part of Hodder & Stoughton Limited
An Hachette Company

The authorized representative in the EEA is Hachette Ireland,
8 Castlecourt Centre, Dublin 15, D15 TP3, Ireland (email: infohbgi.ie)

For Ellie and Phoebe

Contents

Foreword

Living with a fatiguing health condition such as ME, CFS, fibromyalgia or Long Covid is deeply challenging on multiple levels. We are living in a time when there is a marked increase in the numbers of people living with these sorts of conditions. Part of the lived experience challenge is that the mechanisms causing and driving these conditions are poorly understood and are therefore not easily treated. This leaves people with both the challenge of managing the day-to-day difficulties the condition presents, as well as the psychological implications of living with uncertainty and a sense of powerlessness. In this context, it is vital that support is available to resource sufferers with self-management methods that can be implemented in everyday life, combined with an invitation to engage in a deep dive personal exploration oriented towards cultivating a wise and compassionate engagement with this unwanted visitor.

In this remarkable book, Fiona McKechnie is a wonderfully skilful guide exploring the interface between long-term fatigue-based health conditions and training in mindfulness. She is hugely well placed to be a guide in this area. What you hold in your hands is based on more than two decades of clinical practice dedicated to this interface, combined with more than three decades of personal engagement in mindfulness practice and study, including completing a Master's in Mindfulness-based Approaches with my team at Bangor University. You can therefore be confident that the approach and methodologies that you will read about in this book have been well thought through and thoroughly tested, with invaluable lived experience input from the hundreds of people who have engaged with Fiona in her mindfulness courses over the years. Their voices, stories, discoveries and wisdom shine through the pages.

Fiona is a pioneer who has gone ahead and explored the terrain and has generously come back to offer us what she has discovered, in a way that is digestible and engaging. She skilfully details the subtlety of the implications of a mindful approach to living with health challenges. A key question that mindfulness will support an experiential engagement with is: 'How am I in relationship with this illness, with this unwanted visitor?' This is a critical question because how we orient to our experience shapes our perspective, which in turn shapes our lived experience. We generally cannot choose the cards we are dealt in life, but if we are resourced through well-delivered training in mindfulness, we can discover how to wisely orient towards what is showing up in our lives. Mindfulness supports us to shift from an aversive reactive relationship to our lived reality,[1] to a relationship characterized by a sustained friendly, interested engagement in lived reality. This shift in perspective transforms how we engage, so shaping the daily choices we make, which in turn can have profoundly transformative effects, both in relation to the health challenge itself, and in relation to the entirety of our life. In this way, living with what is very understandably experienced as 'unwanted' can turn out to be a doorway into a deeper understanding of life, and into connection with what feels most important and valued to us. In brief, a depth mindful, compassionate engagement with difficult life experience can be a catalyst to wisdom.

What you hold in your hand is a key that unlocks access to these insights and transformations, and to the inner resources that each participant engaging with these programmes already has within them. Fiona unpacks the particularities of the various lived challenges that come with fatigue-based health conditions, and the processes that underpin them. She then links these to how elements of the mindfulness curriculum offer wise and compassionate ways of engaging with these difficulties, including accessible presentations of the theoretical principles underpinning these, and the practicalities of teaching them to others.

The treasures within the book will be particularly valuable to mindfulness-based programme teachers who are either explicitly teaching this population; or are finding (which is commonly the case) that significant numbers of individuals with these kinds of long-term health conditions are joining regular courses, and the teacher wants to tailor elements of the delivery to make the application of the learning to the health condition clearer. As well as discovering how to fine tune established mindfulness-based programme curriculums to this population, you will find invaluable evidence-based pointers on how to proactively engage with the process of implementing this work in your clinical context, and how to develop a mindfulness-based fatigue and pain management service. The process of training as an MBP teacher both generally and for this population is also addressed. The book will also be helpful as a guide for people living with fatigue-based conditions if there isn't a taught course available to attend. In practice though, the learning tends to be deeper and more enduring when it takes place in the context of support from a clear programme structure, with a skilled teacher, and with a group of fellow participants to co-journey with.

---

1   Aversion is a profoundly natural and understandable reaction to living with ongoing and unexplained fatigue and pain, hence the importance of embedding all these teachings in kindness and compassion.

This great book explores both the philosophical underpinnings to a mindfulness-based approach to life's challenges, as well as offering practical guidance on how to bring these into being. Fiona's sustained leadership and development of mindfulness services for people with fatigue-based health challenges, coupled with her own depth engagement with mindfulness practices and teachings, put her in a unique position to guide us in this area. I am deeply confident that if the wisdom in this book is brought to life in the practice of teaching mindfulness-based courses for people with fatigue-based health challenges, it will transform the lives of people who participate. I unreservedly commend it to you.

Professor Rebecca Crane, PhD, Director,
Centre for Mindfulness Research and Practice, Bangor University

Foreword

I first met Fiona in 2012 when I was her tutor on the Master's in Mindfulness-based Approaches at Bangor University. I remember her bright enthusiasm and infectious sense of humour. Since that time, we have stayed in touch through supervision and I have witnessed her dedication to create a mindfulness-based approach to fatigue within the Bristol ME/CFS service. I know that she was inspired by Trish Bartley's adaptation of MBCT for depression for cancer patients. As you will read in these pages, effective formulation and adaptation are at the heart of Fiona's work. The lived experience of patients is front and centre here both in terms of listening, recording and responding to patient feedback and also in encouraging patients to continue their involvement in the project.

And now after helping hundreds of patients, Fiona has written this book to make her approach more widely available to other clinicians. At a time when Long Covid is increasing worldwide, such an approach is more needed than ever before.

I am delighted that, with this book, the sustained commitment Fiona and her colleagues show in this crucial field of management of fatigue will be recognized and celebrated more widely. This step-by-step description of a mindfulness-based approach to ME/CFS will enable more clinicians and teachers to offer these tools to those suffering from fatigue in its many forms more confidently and effectively.

Dh Taravajra, LLM, MA in Mindfulness-Based Approaches, Bangor University, Senior trainer in MBCT and MBSR, Centre for Mindfulness Research and Practice, Bangor, Mindfulness Network and Sussex Mindfulness Centre

Acknowledgements

This book is an amalgamation of thoughts, conversations and connections. Some of it was written from scratch, some from talks and workshops I've run, and some from service evaluations and feedback forms. I wrote it while working full time in an expanding team and as a single parent. The main thing that kept me going was the participant stories and reflections, their ongoing commitment to mindfulness practice and the support they give to not only each other but also those of us working in a field where there are no easy answers or quick results. The enthusiasm for the project was heartening and Rhonda Knight and Sarah Nearney kept spurring me on with their thoughts and ideas as well as their written sections. This book would not have happened without them. The following are people I would like to acknowledge for their role in the past 12 years of developing this programme.

Aysha Adrissi, psychology assistant, and Susanne Davis, MSc student, who interviewed and ran focus groups for participants, were pivotal in organizing the feedback and thoughts of the participants. Their gentle intelligence meant we have been able to reflect the thoughts and feelings of people who go through the course and have developed it based on this work.

The team in North Bristol NHS Trust, particularly Hazel O'Dowd, my head of service, clinical supervisor and friend, who let me try mindfulness out and supported the development of the programme; Peter Gladwell, who has now also trained as a mindfulness teacher and been instrumental in maintaining the integrity of the programme and its place in the department through business plans and staffing as well as his skilful practice; Sarah Horne for her involvement at the start, support in my Master's funding application and ongoing friendship and wisdom; Crispin Barker for his joyful development of embodied contemplative practice in our clinical work; Beverly Knops (now at Vitality 360) for her friendship and pragmatism with absolute commitment to the patients and good practice; and the rest of the team for their commitment to the work we do as well as being a delightful and interesting bunch of colleagues.

In the ME and pain world, Kirsty Northcott, OT and team lead in Devon, has been a longstanding source of knowledge and understanding, and we have shared our development of mindfulness-based therapy for fatigue as well as a common interest in wild swimming. Also, Christina Surawy at the Oxford Mindfulness Centre for supervision whilst setting up the programme and the group we had with Kate Rimes and other mindfulness teachers interested in ME/CFS.

The team at the Centre for Mindfulness Research and Practice, particularly Vanessa Hope, Taravajra, Trish Bartley and Rebecca Crane, have been pivotal in the development of my practice while I studied the MSc in Mindfulness-based Approaches and through ongoing connection via the mindfulness network. Taravajra has been particularly important through ongoing supervision, his long-term view of what I am doing and how it has unfolded, and his pointing out the particularities of the approach that was emerging in the fatigue group. Through him I have felt ongoing connection to the wider mindfulness world. Trish Bartley was my tutor on the MSc and I found her grounded and fiercely compassionate teaching resonant. Her book on mindfulness for cancer is very clear and inspired me to be as clear as I could in sharing the thinking and processes of the fatigue course. Rebecca Crane gently suggested over several years that I needed to share some of this in some way and has provided a very generous foreword.

Other influences inspire my personal meditation practice. I'd particularly like to acknowledge the Foundation for the Preservation of the Mahayana Tradition (FPMT) and Lama Zopa where my practice started in Dharamsala in 1992; the Insight Meditation Society teachings, particularly Joseph Goldstein and Sharon Salzburg; and Gaia House, particularly Christina Feldman, Martine Batchelor, Jenny Wilks, Suvaco and Yanai Postelnik. Reggie Ray and the dharma ocean embodied practices were a significant development in my personal practice as well as influence on my teaching and the development of this programme. The friendships I found in that circle are ongoing nourishment and support. Yoga teachers Claire Smedley and Naomi Seager have been important to my ongoing practice; Mark Walsh's work on embodied yoga principles clarified bridging the contemplative into the day to day. More recently I have engaged with Guy Burgs and the art of meditation, whose integrity and clarity I currently appreciate.

The Tibetan Vajrayana practice of using life's challenges to develop wisdom and compassion has been a theme I have maintained since the beginning of my relationship with meditation, and I'd like to acknowledge my dearest late friend Lucy Porter with whom I shared this experience on our travels and house share and whose BS detector was strong and hilarious. From this I have the gentle friendship of Venerable Kassapo and Avikara Vajra Rimpoche of the Sakya tradition and I still practise the 'upside down meta bavana'.

Other people to acknowledge are Simon Barnes, my partner in crime travelling up to Bangor for four years and his humorous approach to our endeavours; and Julia Wallond for shared teaching and practice and the development of the work for the National Centre for Integrative Medicine. An important figure for several years was Chris Bowles, who I met via our local mindfulness network and with whom I ran mindfulness-based courses within local primary mental health, Oasis Talk and then the National Centre for Integrative Medicine. She trained with Bangor and then Breathworks, and we supported each other in running both Breathworks and MBSR courses, learning and maintaining the integrity of each curriculum.

The team at Jessica Kingsley Publishers for going with this project and gently easing me into maintaining deadlines, and particularly Peter the copyeditor who had the thankless task of making some of my rambling sentences make sense. While writing this book at times I became very stuck and fearful of how it may be received. I had two coaches through this, Eve Russel who helped me keep the vision and the practical management of the task with timely check ins and Jane Evans who helped me with my fears and beliefs about what I was doing.

While I have a long-standing meditation and yoga practice, offering mindfulness as a course in this way would not have come about without finding Nigel Wellings and Philippa Vick teaching the eight-week course down the road in Bath. I like to blame Nigel and Philippa for the whole enterprise because if they had not done it so well and offered such an interesting and life-changing (as well as enjoyable) course, I'm not sure I would have gone ahead. They remain in my life as dear teachers and an inspiration with their ongoing gatherings.

I am very lucky to have a great group of friends to share life's joys and sorrows, friends who leave cakes outside my back door; insist we go on a trip to the beach; have long and wide-ranging Whatsapp group conversations with; sort my tomato plants out; know when what is needed is a river swim and a bag of crisps or a long walk where we get utterly lost while in deep conversation instead of map reading; or a bottle of wine and good cheese by a fire with salacious jokes, politics and poetry.

Finally, I would like to acknowledge my daughters and mother who have lived with me disappearing off on retreats and into my study to write my MSc and then this book. They have not just put up with it but have been actively encouraging me to continue with work that is personally meaningful and hopefully helpful to others.

Fiona McKechnie, Wiltshire

Chapter 1

Introduction

> This mindfulness programme is a co-creation between therapists and patients based in best mindfulness practice and current models of care for fatigue and pain, including patient co-delivery.

Mindfulness-based programmes merge 'contemplative teaching and meditative practice [with] Western scientific method, medicine, and psychology' (Crane 2017a). To do this requires an understanding of the practices, their pedagogy and a detailed and specialist knowledge of the particularities or specific vulnerabilities of the people we help (Crane, Karunavira and Griffith 2021). This book endeavours to show how a mindfulness-based approach can support living with a fatiguing condition.

> 'It wasn't just the skills or the tricks and the reminders, the anchors and all those techniques, the pacing and things like that. But it was also that I learnt a lot about myself... I learnt that I'm much stronger than I sometimes think I am. But...I'm also quite fragile...it's a real juxtaposition, in being able to find that balance. But actually going to the classes and being involved in a group allowed me to see what others were going through. And I was able to compare myself... But then also not to feel guilty. Or feel that I shouldn't be there. So it was good for me to be kind to myself... Yeah, I think, that was probably one of the biggest things that I've learnt.' (Patient quote)

The medical answer to fatigue is not straightforward, and there is little understanding of why fatigue affects so many to the extent it does. Managing fatigue can feel difficult and isolating, and despite recommendations to recognize and diagnose within months, health practitioners and others are often sceptical of the illness and people are often waiting years for a diagnosis (Chew-Graham et al. 2010; NICE 2021c). Within the chronic fatigue specialism there has been controversy in defining and understanding these conditions (Sharp and Greco 2019; Weir and Speight 2021). Treatments have been contested, and recently cognitive behavioural therapy (CBT) and graded exercise therapy (GET) have been changed within the NICE guidance (NICE 2021c). There is no definitive treatment where it is even available. Similar challenges are being reported amongst those with Long Covid.

There is a significant research base to mindfulness-based approaches concluding that mindfulness-based therapies are effective for a variety of psychological problems, particularly reducing anxiety, depression and stress (Khoury et al. 2013; NICE 2022). There are small studies that have examined the efficacy and experience of mindfulness in myalgic encephalomyelitis/chronic fatigue syndrome (ME/CFS) (O'Dowd and Griffith 2022; Rimes and Wingrove 2013; Surawy, Roberts and Silver 2005), and a review of mind-body interventions in ME/CFS concluded:

> Fatigue severity, anxiety/depression and physical and mental functioning were shown to be improved in patients receiving MBIs (Mind body interventions). However, small sample sizes, heterogeneous diagnostic criteria, and a high risk of bias may challenge this result. Further research using standardized outcomes would help advance the field. (Khanpour Ardestani et al. 2021)

The clinical evidence base for using this approach in fatigue is primarily based on supported self-management as analysed in current NICE guidance (NICE 2021a, 2021b, 2021c) as well as on the work with the thousands of people our services have helped. The mindfulness approach shared here is a synthesis of supported self-management and mindfulness-based group work. Group work means that participants can support each other, and participants will often have prior information on self-management through groups (e.g. pain management programmes). Mindfulness is a way of accessing that knowledge experientially and putting it into practice in the moment. It is also hypothesized that mindfulness supports the struggle that people experience in self-managing, for example the challenge of changing habits and patterns as well as feelings of guilt, shame and loss.

Structure of this book

This book is divided into four parts. Part 1 begins by outlining the current understanding of the health conditions ME/CFS, fibromyalgia and Long Covid. For some (uncertain) reason it seems the body has not recovered from illness, injury or trauma and is in a dysregulated state of protection from internal (e.g. viral) threat or external stressors. This leads to a cluster of symptoms including fatigue, pain and cognitive problems that impact significantly on day-to-day life. A 'mild' form is known to affect the sufferer's ability to work or attend education, and this impact lasts for several years or can be lifelong. Severe forms can see people bedbound needing total care (NICE 2021c). Our multi-disciplinary team of physiotherapists, occupational therapists and psychologists see people when all medically treatable options for the symptoms have been pursued and people have the challenging task of 'living with it'. The team approach is based on supporting the self-management of longer-term fatigue and pain conditions, including ME/CFS, fibromyalgia and Long Covid. The different clinicians overlap core skills and can offer particular expertise according to need. Part 1 considers how underlying processes within a mindfulness-based approach can map onto and support self-management. It also considers how mindfulness can work with specific challenges including cognitive fatigue or 'brain fog'.

Part 2 goes into the specifics of the practices, course themes, intentions and adaptations. My physiotherapy colleagues Peter Gladwell and Sarah Nearney have developed movements and an inquiry process for the course. Sarah was initially a patient volunteer; in 2020 she commenced an MSc in mindfulness-based approaches at Aberdeen University, and we now employ her to work as course therapist/co-facilitator. Peter is both a physiotherapist and mindfulness teacher and is team lead for the Bristol ME/CFS service.

In Part 3, we go on to consider how a mindfulness-based approach can be translated into everyday life including rest, activity and setback management.

Part 4 is a week-by-week breakdown of the mindfulness programme as it is at the time of writing. We use a structure based on a definition of what entails a mindfulness-based intervention (MBI), centring on a mindfulness practice with reflection and inquiry, peer support and discussion of home practice, a themed discussion and then more practice rather than following a rigid timetable (Kuyken et al. 2021; Santorelli et al. 2017). Rhonda Knight kept a journal on her first course and then joined us as a patient volunteer and has continued to journal over the years. She shares her insights and reflections on the programme week by week and documents her journey 'From doing to being'.

Throughout the book are case illustrations with significantly changed features, so that they are not identifiable to a specific person. This was easy to do as the experience of the conditions are so similar across a disparate range of people, ages, backgrounds and experiences. The quotes from patients are from anonymized transcripts compiled by Aysha Adrissi and Susanne Davis from focus groups and interviews.

Finally, training, supervision and staff development is considered as well as current resources.

Development and implementation

There has been work looking at the implementation of mindfulness, particularly mindfulness-based cognitive therapy (MBCT), which is recommended in the NICE guidelines for depression. The ASPIRE study (Crane et al. 2021; Rycroft-Malone et al. 2017) found the successful creation and maintenance of an MBCT service have the following common characteristics:

- 'Making it fit' the service you are working within
- Evaluating the service and learning from it
- Creating networks and building a culture
- Building a team to deliver
- Getting top-down buy-in
- Creating a fit-for-purpose structure/governance
- Nourishing and sustaining yourselves and your colleagues.

The ASPIRE project fits very much with our experience and the way we have embedded the approach within the service and have developed ourselves and our team as it progressed.

Developing a specific programme

I started delivering a mindfulness-based course in 2011 following conversations with patients who had completed fatigue and pain management programmes, some of whom had found mindfulness, meditation and other practices to be helpful, and some who felt they needed more support. I had a longstanding meditation and yoga practice (since 1990) and had come across MBCT in the book *The Mindful Way Through Depression* (Williams et al. 2007) and in 2009 attended a course for myself (Bath and Bristol Mindfulness course). From running a few sessions and embarking on further training that resulted in a six-year training programme and an MSc at Bangor University, with supervision from Christina Surawy at the Oxford Mindfulness Centre, a specific course for people with fatigue and pain, particularly ME/CFS and fibromyalgia (FMS), has developed over the years, and recently people with Long Covid have started to join.

The programme is based on the published mindfulness-based programmes with adaptations to some of the practices and exercises. As it is delivered within a self-management programme there are cultural facets that support the learning and experience. The following factors have been remarked upon by participants and facilitators:

- The programmes are run by personnel who have an understanding of the condition, including diagnostic processes and the symptoms, and are aware of the impact of these health conditions on day-to-day life and the huge disruption to careers, family life and ambitions.
- People with a lived experience are part of the programme delivery.
- There is a shared understanding and commonality of experience between the participants, who may not have the same diagnosis but do have similar health experiences.
- The sessions are paced to allow participants to experiment with

movement and postural changes that enable their participation in the course. Breaks, pauses and repetition support varying and fluctuating symptoms, including cognitive challenges.

- Practices can be graded so that people find their own way with them and can adapt them if they have symptom exacerbation.
- The in-room sessions and online sessions are managed to support access: in the room, there are different types of chairs, mats and cushions and footstools; online, there is no rule to have the camera on; people can take breaks when they need to; there is a protected break in both sessions; sessions start and finish on time; and people can come late and leave early and are welcomed to do as best they can.
- Didactic information is kept to a minimum, and the emphasis is on practice and inquiry with each session having a focus or intention, as per the mindfulness-based stress reduction (MBSR) programme (Santorelli et al. 2017).

Making a strong case

During the development stage, we collected measurements using our standard service measures and fed outcomes back to the service and also obtained feedback from both patients and colleagues. While I am currently employed entirely within the ME/CFS service, I have worked within pain management and maintain connections with the team and supervise the occupational therapists in pain management. Physiotherapy and psychology colleagues also work across both services, so there is a cohesiveness of culture and understanding that is embedded within the mindfulness-based programme. There is a constant referral into the group with a low non-attendance rate, to the extent that we are now running approximately six groups a year with 12–15 participants plus monthly follow-up sessions attended by approximately 20–30 people. Others are seen individually. Figure 1.1 shows the relationships between the pain management, ME and Long Covid services and where the mindfulness-based programme sits.

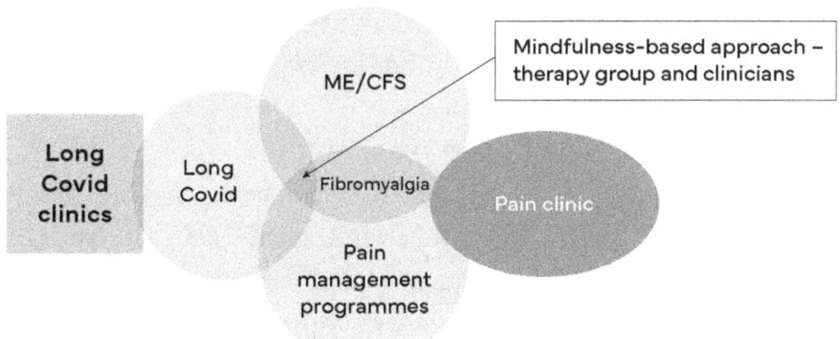

Figure 1.1 Relationship between services and mindfulness-based location

The development of the course has been supported by management and in 2019 led to a specific post of mindfulness-based therapist to coordinate this part of the service while being embedded within the wider teams. Other teachers, training, supervision and administrative support are also resourced.

Theoretical background and curriculum choices

This programme is based on published mindfulness programmes: the MBCT courses for depression (Williams et al. 2007) and cancer (Bartley 2011), MBSR (Kabat-Zinn 2013; Santorelli et al. 2017) and is also influenced by Breathworks mindfulness for health (Burch and Penman 2013). The course was run for several years using the MBCT format with some adaptations for ME/CFS (Rimes and Wingrove 2013; Surawy et al. 2005). This was influenced by training at Bangor University specifically with Trish Bartley with supervision from Christina Surawy (who started MBCT for ME/CFS at the Oxford Mindfulness Centre), then ongoing supervision from Taravajra (also an MBCT teacher at Bangor University and the Sussex Mindfulness Centre). There was also an opportunity to co-run MBSR and Breathworks courses with Chris Bowles (MBSR and Breathworks teacher) within the Bristol pain management and primary mental health services as well as MBCT for cancer courses with the National Centre for Integrative Medicine and the Penny Brohn Centre.

The MBCT, Breathworks and MBSR curricula were used in a 'pure' way intentionally to maintain the integrity of those courses that had been designed with extensive research, thought and evaluation. This was our training ground in the approach, so we became immersed in the programme as designed rather than trying to change things in the first instance. From using these programmes over a few years, and discussion within supervision structures, we identified that there were specific adaptations we were using for particular reasons within the service. The changes emerged from:

- developments and understanding of theoretical models of pain and fatigue and post-viral conditions
- the reported experiences of a reflective team and the participants
- our own developing and 'live' mindfulness practice.

DEVELOPING MODELS OF HEALTH AND THERAPY

As the ME/CFS and pain field developed over the years, and a dysregulation model to understand ME/CFS, fibromyalgia and chronic pain emerged (BACME 2021; Clark et al. 2019; Clauw 2010; Morris et al. 2019; Nijs et al. 2012) alongside knowledge of trauma-informed approaches (Porges 2007; van der Kolk 2014), the mindfulness field was also developing along trauma and neurobiologically informed lines (Chew-Graham et al. 2010; Treleaven 2018; van Dam et al. 2018).

These approaches are increasingly becoming mainstream and inform the lens through which both clinicians and participants view their experiences.

CO-CREATING THE PROGRAMME WITH PARTICIPANTS

We have intentionally used a bottom-up practice-based approach in the development of the programme, listening carefully to patients and bringing their experience of using mindfulness-based practices and approaches into the delivery and the style and content of the programme within the context of the services. This is supported by long-term service-user involvement and a programme of trained lay tutors with lived experience within the pain management service. The mindfulness-based courses have been extremely fortunate to have dedicated volunteers to support patients and be part of our team. They have informed both the content and delivery by sharing their practice and being available as a sounding board to discuss how the programme was developing and offer ideas and perspective as well as weekly practical involvement and delivery of the courses. The outcomes from the programme have shown consistent improvements in anxiety, depression and pain as well as improved quality of life. Satisfaction in the programme has been high.

CLINICIAN PERSONAL PRACTICE

The need for personal practice is a requirement of teaching mindfulness (UK Network of Mindfulness Teacher Training Organisations 2015), and experience in my own practice has fed into the programme, including hatha yoga teacher training and immersion in insight practices and retreats as well as the somatic meditation protocols based on Tibetan Buddhism developed by Reginald Ray (Ray 2016). This resonated with developments such as trauma-informed practice, and the mindfulness course and practices started to adapt and reflect some of these influences. The course varied from one-and-a-half to two-hour sessions and were either weekly or fortnightly, or sometimes a varying pattern based on pragmatic decisions (room bookings, therapist availability, etc.).

CHANGES MADE

The changes made were discussed in detail with patient volunteers as well as the clinical team. Participants have consented for quotes from the focus groups and questionnaires to be used throughout this guide to highlight the experience of individuals learning mindfulness to manage their lives with a chronically fatiguing health condition. Their willingness to work in this way is inspiring and very much informs the groups and our work.

The course's skeleton is mindfulness-based cognitive therapy (Bartley 2011; Rimes and Wingrove 2013; Segal, Williams and Teasdale 2013) with adaptations for this group of people who live with a particular pattern of symptoms and have been through a process of diagnosis and a service that uses a self-management approach. The challenges that arise from both living with the condition and the self-management approach are addressed throughout the course and detailed in subsequent chapters. The basis of the changes are detailed throughout the book and the specifics are considered in Part 4. The changes are often change of nuance or application rather than a radical change.

- *Changes to format*: The format is not hugely changed from an MBCT course, but from the evaluation we moved to definitely running on a fortnightly basis and limited the time to two hours. An all-day session has not been trialled; on reflection and discussion, it is likely this would exclude too many participants as well as being a logistical challenge within a busy clinic.
- *Changes to content*: As a mindfulness-based approach, the practice and experiential learning are central; however, there are particular changes based on understanding of the condition, particularly living with post-exertional symptom exacerbation (or malaise) which leads to the 'boom-and-bust' nature of the conditions and the specific challenge of setbacks.
- *Changes to practices*: Practices were simplified based on: analysis of reflective logs during a course; discussion with participants in individual appointments after each group; and in the monthly follow-on sessions. Theoretical understanding and knowledge (e.g. dysregulation, neurobi-ology, cognitive challenges with attention, etc.) underpin each practice and the flow of practices following a format that builds week to week – from grounding and body awareness in the body scan; using the short pauses (breathing spaces) to ground and check in; and then the practices were used to notice difficulty by practising the self-care and skills taught earlier in the course, enabling choices and changes to be made.

Explicit emphasis is made of regulating and being able to identify and work with the stress reaction through awareness and movement. The movement practices have been developed to explore alternatives to the boom-and-bust approach to activity by exploring the nourishing and nurturing nature of movement and what is possible if we are curious about the feeling of movement in the body as it is now.

The practices are repetitive, following an almost routine format but with different intentions. This is on purpose, based on the observed clinical need of the population to stop and rest and settle their 'system', and doing this through the body simplifies it and makes it more readily accessible. The cognitive challenges people experience, to the extent that they sometimes say they do not understand words, means that 'feeling in' through movement and a routine and repetition in the practices is helpful, as is the sparce didactic content.

Application and folding into daily life is a significant part of the whole approach. The people we see often have to make huge changes in what and how they do things. Mindfulness provides a way to look at the quality, texture and emotion of activity and find ways of inhabiting new ways of being. My background as an occupational therapist informs this approach and the detail of activity analysis and management required to navigate living with fatiguing conditions.

Follow-on sessions

We run monthly hour-long sessions attended by between 20 and 30 people on video calls. The feedback we have from these sessions is that being with others in a similar boat who have experienced the mindfulness course is of huge benefit. And that boat includes not just the lived experience of the condition, but also the language and culture of the service that diagnosed the condition and provides physiotherapy, occupational and psychological therapies and specific advice on matters such as medication, sleep and diet. Locating the group within the service allows particular follow-up questions relevant to the whole service (e.g. questions about Covid vaccinations were brought to the group in one session). A criticism is that perhaps we are holding them too closely, so it is then difficult for people to pick up community services, and a more autonomous element to the process may need to be considered in the future as well as improving links to some of the excellent local community resources available. Signposting and recommending in emails does not seem to have carry-over as yet and is worthy of further thought.

The pandemic 2020 onwards

The pandemic and lockdowns meant that further changes were made, and the course immediately moved to an online programme. Shorter groups were experimented with, but patient volunteers fed back that two hours remained optimal as that gave more time and opportunity for a longer break. Weekly sessions were also trialled; however, this was too intense, and the fortnightly pattern resumed. All materials were made available online. Practices were re-recorded, and in line with changes made in mindfulness programmes, due to the anxiety and respiratory problems during the pandemic, practices changed to move attention away from the breath to discovering how to anchor in various parts of the body and the environment. At the time of writing, the practices are being reconsidered as the breath has been a powerful focus of meditation and other practices for millennia. The main learning is that the practices need to be 'alive' and contemporary and bear in mind social and cultural changes as well as the needs of each group and participant.

We are now including people with Long Covid who have been through the fatigue service. We have also been able to include more severely affected participants and take up and attendance has overall been exceptionally good. The likelihood is at least 50% of the courses will remain online due to the increased accessibility. The current session plans are assuming online delivery in obvious contrast to how this was initially intended.

There is a need for good-quality research to investigate and refine this programme. One of the intentions of writing and publishing in this format is to collate what we have done so far within one service and to create a resource that could be developed by clinicians and researchers. Interesting questions could be in these areas:

- Does a mindfulness-based programme enhance self-management?
- What enhances rest in people with fatigue syndromes?
- Does mindfulness-based attention training help with brain fog? And if so, what circumstances optimize this?
- What is the experience of engaging in meaningful and valued activity with a mindful attitude?
- What impact does mindfulness have on quality of life as well as clinical outcomes?

Using the book

This book could be used by mindfulness teachers interested in working with fatigue or find themselves teaching people who are living with a fatiguing health condition, and hopefully there is enough information about the conditions and how mindfulness may be challenging as well as helpful.

Clinicians and therapists working with people who have fatiguing conditions may find understanding more about the mindfulness approach applicable and may be able to use some of the material in their practice. While this isn't designed as a self-help manual, those who live with fatigue may find they can use the material and the guided practices on the website.

A note on language: Subject and personal pronouns

Mindfulness-based therapy is steeped in the practitioner's practice. The current UK standards and training organizations require several years of personal practice before teacher training commences (UK Network of Mindfulness Teacher Training Organisations 2015). The 'inside out group model' (Griffith, Bartley and Crane 2019) unpacks the role of the teacher's mindfulness practice that underpins the group process as the teacher holds and reads the group. This embeds the therapist's personal practice as an anchor for the practitioner as well as a therapeutic medium. Writing about the development of the programme and how the practices are shared includes personal reflections to illustrate the details of how a practice can unfold, so sometimes I am referring to my own practice as well as the 'we' of shared practice and sometimes to 'they' of the participants. This is not always in line with perfect grammar where a consistent subject reads more clearly so it may seem to jump around; however, this is intentional to represent the 'inside out' nature of the programme development.

SUMMARY

The mindfulness for fatigue and pain programme is based on therapists' personal experience of mindfulness theory and practice and clinical experience and knowledge; new knowledge is folded in through discussion and inquiry and evaluated within the team that includes patient experts.

- Adaptations have been made based on observations and practice with participants and detailed feedback using a co-creative process.
- The resulting programme is embedded in published MBCT and MBSR courses with specific changes in emphases in the practices and some session content change.
- The implementation of the programme seems to reflect the experiences documented by the ASPIRE project and has a bottom-up approach with top-down support.
- There is a need for further research to investigate the clinical outcomes and maintain development.

Fatiguing Health Conditions and the Principles of a Mindfulness-Based Approach to Self-Management

This part briefly looks at the health conditions ME/CFS, fibromyalgia and Long Covid and how a mindfulness-based approach may help self-management. We will consider what the conditions are, the way a diagnosis is reached and how the conditions are related in this context. A feature of the fatiguing illnesses is that the core condition is not easily treated. While there are distinct symptoms that are classified as ME/CFS, fibromyalgia and Long Covid, we do not know what the mechanism is for the persistence of the symptoms. The health approach in these conditions is to treat any potential causes of fatigue symptoms (such as sleep problems, menopause, etc.) and then move to a self-management model. While the separate diagnoses are important as each condition has specific features. For the purposes of mindfulness and a course that is more general, a transdiagnostic model is discussed that clusters by symptoms and impact links the conditions. From then on, the conditions are referred to as fatigue syndromes.

Managing a health condition is hard work and challenging. Knowing what we are dealing with is the first step and appreciating that living with a fatigue syndrome is complex and can be seen in layers:

- The illness, its onset and ongoing symptoms and impact.
- The problem that the illness does not have a straightforward remedy and persists, in many cases, for years. And to add to the complexity, it fluctuates.

- It can take a long time to come to a diagnosis and many experience disbelief from health practitioners, employers, friends and family.
- The consequences of the problem. There are health, social and economic consequences both for the individual, their family and the wider community. They do need to be addressed, otherwise the problem can spiral. Tackling the consequences means people feel better, take control, and engage more fully in their lives despite remaining unwell.
- The problem with the solution to the problem. Tackling the consequences takes time, energy and resources (personal resources as well as health and other services): self-management is of itself challenging.
- Reaction. Understandably no one wants any of this, and the reaction is to avoid or fight it causing other problems. Everyone involved reacts – the individual reacts to it, their family, friends and workplaces react to it, health professionals react to it – and this can again compound the problem.

Knowing what we are dealing with, in other words seeing that there is a problem and that problem is complex and that there are ways to approach it, is the first step in a mindfulness-based approach. This part of the book explores 'the problem' using the following questions:

- What are the conditions ME/CFS, fibromyalgia and Long Covid?
- Why are they grouped together in this programme?
- How have we been using mindfulness to help?

Chapter 2

Overview of ME/CFS, Fibromyalgia and Long Covid

- Definition of fatigue
- Prevalence of fatigue syndromes
- Symptoms and diagnosis
- The experience of being diagnosed, referred to a specialist clinic and additional challenges
- Distinguishing between Long Covid, ME/CFS and fibromyalgia – benefits and challenges

Fatigue is a common symptom, most people will relate to it and know what is meant by the term, synonyms of which are tiredness, weariness, exhaustion, overtiredness, drowsiness, somnolence, lethargy, sluggishness, lassitude, and so on. It is a feature of many health conditions, including cancer, stroke, multiple sclerosis (MS), lung disease, rheumatoid arthritis, anxiety, heart failure, and so on. 'Poorly understood' is repeatedly reported when considering the fatiguing elements of these health conditions. Treatments are developed to improve the underlying cause of the condition, and at best this work hopes to improve the fatigue by tackling the underlying disease process. In reality, fatigue is unlikely to be measured (Davis and Walsh 2010; Finsterer and Mahjoub 2014; Swain 2000). There is no medical specialism in fatigue, no hospital department specific to it. ME/CFS clinics are often part of other specialities: neurology and pain management; rheumatology; immunology; psychiatry; and there are some services supported by general physicians or practitioners with special interests.

The fatigue we are talking about here is not tiredness; it is sometimes described as 'malaise', defined in the Merriam-Webster online dictionary as 'an indefinite feeling of debility or lack of health often indicative of or accompanying the onset of an illness'. The malaise fluctuates, often exacerbated after doing something, and is termed post-exertional malaise (PEM) (NICE 2021c). This chapter endeavours to describe the clusters of symptoms that are common to all these conditions and to describe 'post-exertional malaise' in more specific terms.

Prevalence

Population studies around the world report the symptom patterns described above; they are not a feature of certain racial or socioeconomic groups, although more women than men are diagnosed with fibromyalgia and ME/CFS (Hickie 2009; Reeves et al. 2007; Wessely et al. 1997). Millions of people are affected, and by 'affected' we mean daily lives are disrupted, including work and school attendance, with resulting impact on social participation and financial security (Collin et al. 2011; Wurz et al. 2022).

ME/CFS affects approximately 250,000 people in the UK (NICE 2021c); fibromyalgia is estimated to have a worldwide prevalence of 2% (Royal College of Physicians 2022). Long Covid's prevalence is unclear as the diagnostic criteria or range of the condition are not yet known (Alwan and Johnson 2021; Routen et al. 2022).

According to the Office of National Statistics (2022), at the time of writing, of the 2.1 million people (3.3%) of the UK population with self-reported Long Covid, 1.1 million (52%) had Covid at least one year previously and 507,000 (24%) at least two years previously. Long Covid symptoms adversely affected the day-to-day activities of 1.6 million people (76% of those with self-reported Long Covid), with 333,000 (16%) reporting that their ability to undertake their day-to-day activities had been 'limited a lot'. Fatigue continued to be the most common symptom reported as part of individuals' experience of Long Covid (70% of those with self-reported Long Covid), followed by difficulty concentrating (45%), shortness of breath (42%) and muscle ache (42%).

NICE (2021a) observed that the Covid-19 pandemic has created a

> new and emerging condition, which has been described using a variety of terms including 'long COVID', [which] can have a significant effect on people's quality of life. It also presents many challenges when trying to determine the best-practice standards of care based on the current evidence. There is no internationally agreed clinical definition or clear treatment pathway, and there is an evolving evidence base.

ME/CFS and Long Covid both have specific NICE guidance in the UK (NICE 2021a, 2021c). Fibromyalgia comes under chronic pain NICE guidance (2021b), but there is a Royal College of Physicians guide, summarizing the condition as

> a medical condition that causes widespread pain, fatigue and difficulty concentrating. It is multifactorial with neurophysiological, immunological and cognitive elements. It responds poorly to conventional treatments, including medicines and injections. It is best managed with an individualised multi-element support plan. (Royal College of Physicians 2022)

NICE (2021c) classified ME/CFS as mild, moderate, severe and very severe. The 'mild' form will see people struggling to manage full-time work or education and will likely need adjustments to manage to attend. Exercise and mental activity is limited and needs to be managed, whereas 'moderate' often means giving up work, and 50% of people accessing specialist services are likely to lose their job and those in work are likely to be struggling either to maintain hours or find that all they can do is work and all other aspects of life are affected; in other words, they struggle to socialize, do housework and holidays are spent recovering and not engaging in enjoyable activity (Collin et al. 2011). People who are 'moderately' affected may struggle with mobility and use a wheelchair. The group of patients described as having a severe presentation have significant levels of disability requiring personal care and are bedbound. In very severe cases, people could need total care and in some cases are tube fed.

Symptoms and diagnosis

ME/CFS, fibromyalgia and Long Covid are conditions where the fatigue (and, as we will discuss, many other symptoms) predominates, but the mechanism or pathology for what is causing the ongoing symptoms remains elusive. To arrive at a diagnosis, numerous tests are carried out to rule out other causes of the symptoms, but it is not correct to call them 'diagnoses of exclusion'. People coming to the clinics report a consistent set of symptoms and a recurrent pattern to those symptoms. There are also common themes to their history: while in Long Covid the patients are defined by the fact they have had Covid-19 (tested or not), people with ME/CFS have often had a virus or other infection (but not always) and people with fibromyalgia have sometimes had an injury. Many people will have had stress or trauma. Sometimes, though, there is no obvious trigger or precipitating illness or injury, suggesting there is a genetic predisposition.

Table 2.1 lists symptoms reported in clinics around the world. While all these symptoms are classed as fatigue, it is probably more useful to regard the term fatigue (or malaise) as a shorthand to describe the list of symptoms that impact people who come to fatigue clinics. This distinguishes it from tiredness and enables the clinics to focus on those with a particular cluster of disabling symptoms. People don't need to have all the symptoms to be diagnosed, and everyone will have their own specific cluster that may change over time. Clarifying what are the common symptoms does several things:

- It groups the symptoms so people understand that we are not talking only about fatigue. If they have had appropriate tests, then we can consider that the multiple symptoms they experience are part of the same syndrome rather than the result of a host of conditions. For example, the cognitive problems some experience can mean they are worrying about dementia. Asking about this symptom and its impact and providing information can be hugely relieving. (See chapter 7 for more details.)

- Identifying the symptoms means that any symptomatic relief that can be offered can be investigated and trialled; for example, medication for sleep, dietary advice and support for IBS symptoms; postural tachycardia syndrome (POTS) symptoms can be treated, and so on (NICE 2021a, 2021b, 2021c).

- Knowing the shape and pattern of the condition is important as other health problems can arise and need to be identified and treated accordingly. For example, I had a patient who had severe and prolonged bouts of tachycardia and arrythmia requiring visits to hospital – she saw it as part of ME/CFS; however, this was very different to the palpitations described by people with ME/CFS, and she eventually had a cardiac diagnosis and treatment as well as ME/CFS.

Table 2.1 'Fatigue' symptoms

Common symptoms	Less common symptoms
Fatigue, exhaustion, weakness	Sore throat, tender glands
Pain: joints, muscles, headache; gastric; chest	Dizziness
Unrefreshing sleep	Poor balance
Too much/too little sleep	Nausea
'Brain fog', e.g. concentration problems	Sensitivity: noise, light, smells, food
Memory problems	Reduced tolerance to alcohol
Post-exertional malaise	Palpitations
Flu-like symptoms	Pins and needles, twitches
Breathlessness	IBS symptoms

Background to a diagnosis and referral to a specialist clinic

Before presenting for a diagnosis, most people will have experienced a number of challenges, and as clinicians in this field appreciating this context and potential distress is important (Reeves et al. 2007). A typical history has various stages to it:

- An injury or infection (bacterial or viral); often serious and very debilitating at the time.
- A period of stress either before, during or after the infection (which in some cases is the viral infection; for example, contracting Covid in a lockdown is very challenging whether or not you were admitted to

hospital; other examples are contracting a tropical disease and then being in isolation; being resuscitated with sepsis, etc.). Or a period of social or work-related stress, not attached to the precipitating illness.

- A protracted recovery where you think you will be getting better soon so keep doing things, only to be knocked back and have longstanding symptoms. (Going back to work after Covid or glandular fever to find you cannot manage is a very common picture in anecdotal clinical practice.)
- A series of investigations; for some this can include internal investigations (e.g. endoscopies), CT and MRI scans, etc.
- Often being told there is nothing medically wrong but being offered no help and then the individual must keep asking for a referral, support with benefits, etc. (Pilkington et al. 2020).
- Being scared that some of the symptoms (e.g. brain fog) are another condition, perhaps dementia. Note that some people have a huge change in cognitive function (e.g. university lecturers who can no longer read).
- Either being off work for a long time or only just coping (and having no social life) and the resulting loss in income and social connection.
- Having tried different medications, including pain killers and anti-depressants, often at best to little or no effect, or at worst with an adverse reaction or unacceptable side-effects.

Additional challenges some people experience:

- a background of trauma (e.g. childhood trauma) (de Venter et al. 2017; Espeleta et al. 2020; Heim et al. 2009)
- medical practitioners, as well as employers, family members and friends, who 'don't believe' in ME/CFS/fibromyalgia (Chew-Graham et al. 2010); we are also hearing this from some Long Covid people
- media articles that have 'views' and 'advice'; these are often single-person reports with confusing messages about what helps (e.g. exercise and diet information is wide-ranging and contradictory)
- workplace sickness measures
- poverty
- being a carer for a child, partner or parent.

Distinguishing different conditions

There is a case made by some for clarifying the differences between the conditions as they have distinguishing features (e.g. Moghimi et al. 2021). Broadly speaking, people with fibromyalgia have pain as the most predominant symptom; people with ME/CFS have post-exertional and cognitive fatigue;

and people with Long Covid are distinguished by becoming unwell after contracting Covid-19. Long Covid is slightly more complex because this label can cover a host of problems resulting from the Covid virus (Rivas-Vazquez et al. 2022). For the purposes of this book, we are focusing on those where there is no observable pathology and the predominant symptom is 'fatigue' (i.e. a cluster of symptoms listed in Table 2.1) that has been experienced for six months or more and is impeding participation in usual activity.

Ongoing research, particularly into ME/CFS and Long Covid, will hopefully reveal more complex understanding of the mechanisms of this illness and improve treatment options. In terms of helping people manage these health conditions, there are similarities in both symptoms and experience that enable the use of a pragmatic transdiagnostic approach. The work on centralized pain (Clauw 2010) describes a dysregulated nervous system that affects the body's ability to regulate and seems to describe people's experience with these health conditions.

SUMMARY

- Fatigue is often referred to in medical research and texts as 'poorly understood' and is rarely treated directly.
- ME/CFS, fibromyalgia and Long Covid are defined as separate conditions and have their own NICE guidance.
- While other conditions are excluded, these are not diagnoses of exclusion as there are clear and typical symptoms exacerbated by exertion.
- The process of diagnosis is often protracted and exacerbates the distress and challenge people experience.
- The social status of these conditions can increase suffering through disbelief. This was highlighted in the workplace by the TUC's March 2023 report (www.tuc.org.uk/sites/default/files/2023-03/LongCovidatWork23.pdf).
- Early life and ongoing adversity and social exclusion can compound the challenge.
- Covid-19 may be an opportunity as research is ongoing.

Chapter 3

Pragmatic Transdiagnostic Understanding of ME/CFS, Fibromyalgia and Long Covid

- Transdiagnostic understanding
- Metaphors and models to aid understanding and planning therapy
- Consequences – the 'boom-and-bust' pattern
- Assessing the condition and the impact
- Starting to address consequences

This chapter considers a pragmatic transdiagnostic understanding of the conditions people present with despite specific diagnoses. As therapists, we tend to use information that can help in the rehabilitative work we do and will update models and explanations as evidence is presented. This particular model has been found useful by people living with fatigue as it:

- explains why the symptoms are so wide-ranging
- is easy to explain to friends and family
- offers a place to start in taking control of what can feel like an overwhelming situation.

What it doesn't do is explain why some people contract the condition or what its underlying mechanism may be.

A theory is emerging within clinical practice and has been summarized by the ME Clinicians Association (BACME). The numerous yet inconclusive research trials suggest that the symptoms in the fatiguing conditions are a dysregulation of the body's homeostatic system, triggered by infections and/or stressful or traumatic experiences (BACME 2021). What we could call the body's 'protective system' becomes activated whether dealing with an infection or another threat. This system includes the autonomic nervous system and the immune system, which are interlinked and activated under stress or infection. Activation leads to physiological and behavioural changes to maximize healing and enable recovery while protecting the body from threats at a time of vulnerability. Additionally, the activation of the hypothalamic-pituitary-adrenal (HPA) axis in response to stress can in turn lead to immune responses (felt as sore throats and tender glands, reduced concentration, etc.). In post-viral states, it is observed that once the infection has stopped, the body seems to be over-responsive to benign input (e.g. excessively raised heart rate going up the stairs) as though there was something to be 'fought off', hence flu-like symptoms such as heavy limbs and brain fog. It is unclear what the mechanism is to this dysregulation. Clark et al. (2019) describe this phenomenon:

> ...while certain events may represent an initial hit, once this has been removed the consequences may well persist in altered systems regulation. In this way, the key pathology which underpins CFS is potentially best understood in computational terms as resulting from altered messages passing amongst homeostatic networks. Indeed, it is a curious observation that much of what has been shown in the literature can be described as a failure of such networks to regulate themselves.

Having an infection and longer-term symptoms that are not easily treated are in themselves stressful, so there can be a negative cycle that exacerbates and perpetuates the condition.

Pain research suggests similar patterning, and 'Hypersensitivity (termed "central and peripheral sensitisation") of the nervous system to external stimuli can explain many of the sensory symptoms associated with FMS' (Royal College of Physicians 2022).

The complexity of this is underlined by the fact that some people do not have a defined trigger but have a cluster and pattern of symptoms and responses that can be classified as ME/CFS or fibromyalgia. This suggests there could be a genetic component to these conditions.

Dysregulation – an alarm-system model

These metaphors are not perfect. In fact any model has its flaws; as cited by Box and Draper (1987), 'Essentially all models are wrong, but some are useful.' However, shared models can go some way to explaining people's experience and are a starting point for developing a shared understanding.

Finding a workable concept

Without a workable conceptualization of fatigue syndromes there can be uncertainty that leads to a feeling of overwhelm in both patients and clinicians (Jason et al. 2015; Yorkston et al. 2010). How do we work with this in a practical and helpful way? Developing a shared understanding that enables some control of the situation can be useful. As clinicians, we have to be aware that the dysregulation model will change over time, and while so far there is some evidence to support this model, as new information comes in we will need to refine or discard the model (Popper 2005).

Metaphor – a faulty alarm system

A metaphor that can help articulate these complex physiological processes is of an alarm system (e.g. fire alarm) that is set off initially by smoke, but once the smoke has gone it can keep being set off for no apparent reason. The reason there are no clear physiological markers could be that this is a normal, healthy response, but it is happening at inappropriate times and to an excessive degree. Another metaphor is to see the symptoms as a software problem as opposed to a hardware problem – a lot of computer problems would not show up if we scanned the hard drive, rather it is due to some of the processing and communication between the systems.

These metaphors are not perfect, but they go some way to explaining people's experience and are a starting point for developing a shared understanding. They make sense of post-exertional malaise – people report being able to do something but then being hit by symptoms. The alarm model would see that when we do something we are engaging the whole body, nervous system, endocrine system, musculo-skeletal system, cardiovascular system, and so on; in other words, the whole body is involved and is aware that 'something' (BACME 2021; Clark et al. 2019) is happening; however, the communication between the systems becomes akin to an emergency, so the protective elements of the body come on board. These increase heart rate, circulation and autonomic activity, readying the body for action in a reactive pattern (fight/flight). This means other physiological systems that allow us to be more reflective and responsive in a sustaining way cannot easily be engaged. This is exhausting and significantly disrupts sleep and activity patterns. The anxiety response is understandable when the body is in this reactive state, and anxiety understandably exacerbates the sense of 'emergency' in the system. Some patients in clinical practice report going into a 'freeze' state (Porges 2007).

Post-exertional symptoms' effect on activity

Symptoms often fluctuate and people experience better days and worse days in a cycle (see Figure 3.1).

The cycle shown in Figure 3.1 can happen over a few hours, days or weeks. A lot of people report that they feel the repercussions of exertion two to three days after the event. Often, the recovery period is longer than the period of exertion, which means it is very disruptive and frequently distressing to manage and communicate. This pattern of post-exertional malaise, sometimes called the 'boom-and-bust' pattern (see Figure 3.2), is recognized as a key feature of ME/CFS and is also seen in Long Covid, fibromyalgia and other persistent pain and neurological conditions, as well as cancer-related fatigue (Barhorst et al. 2022; Stussman et al. 2020; Twomey et al. 2020).

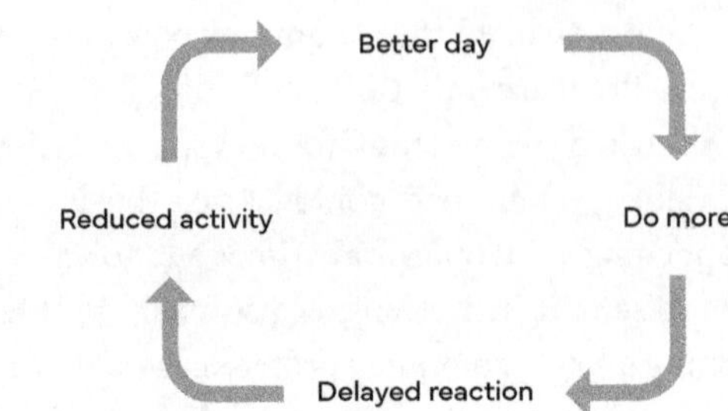

Figure 3.1 *Activity cycle in response to symptoms*

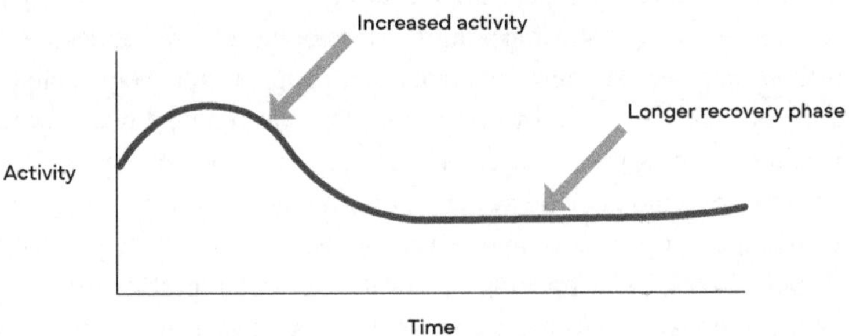

Figure 3.2 *Boom-and-bust pattern of activity*

Impact on daily life

Cognitive symptoms can be as disruptive as physical symptoms, with people struggling to read or use screens for more than a few minutes at a time and experiencing aches and flu-like symptoms as well as fatigue following mental activity as much as physical. Some need to consider how many times they can go up and down stairs or take their children to school. They can become dependent on others not just for practical matters, but also for managing finances and communication.

Making a start – mapping out the situation

Most people seen in the NHS clinics are struggling to manage work or school with substantial economic and social consequences. Resulting anxiety and depression is unsurprising and can reach a level where treatment is required. Pulling together all the strands of the situation and establishing where to focus initially is part of the assessment. This is a brief overview of what may be covered:

INITIAL ASSESSMENT

Medical

History of current health problems and any other health factors.

Current symptom profile:

- Physical – previous level of function and change that may have occurred, including activity level and frequency, sleep, digestion, sensory faculties.
- Cognitive – previous level of function and change that may have occurred (TV, reading, computer, conversation).

Awareness of post-exertional malaise:

- Expect change in activity levels over a day/week/month. Ask about rest – often, people cannot easily rest or sleep and describe a tired but wired state of exhaustion rather than rest.

Social (home, work, finance, etc.)

Context and impact of past as well as current situation and impact of symptoms on individual circumstances.

Emotional

Vulnerabilities, resilience, impact; possibly ask about earlier trauma/difficulties.

The assessment conversation can be challenging and may be the first time someone tells the whole story and talks about the impact and what may be the next step. This also may be the first time that a health professional readily recognizes that all these 'weird changing symptoms' do actually fit together. The alarm-system metaphor often makes sense and is a huge relief. Then there is a discussion that there is no off-switch, that we must work with this rather than fix it. The first step is to get things stabilized as much as they can be. This is a multi-faceted approach that includes physiological stabilization, but also needs to look at wider factors, such as finance, employment, social life and the impact on mental health.

The following are examples of what may be addressed in the initial meetings:

- Work – may need a letter to summarize for work (e.g. AHP fit note); diagnosis and functional description in support of welfare benefits.
- Sleep – pattern may be very disrupted and some targeted work at establishing a more helpful sleep pattern may be required. May need to work with a physician in use of medication (e.g. amitriptyline can help with sleep and pain).
- Mood – may be depressed and find it hard to set goals and priorities. Again, medication and/or specialist mental health support may be required. However, a level of anxiety and low mood is to be expected and may well be helped by the process of getting some help and support.
- Understanding more about the condition – discussion, leaflets, webinars, seminars, meeting others. How will they best access information? What resources are there? We need to be aware that there is a huge amount of opinion and information that is being navigated; being able to use reliable and respected resources that the clinician and the service have gathered or made is useful for a shared understanding and a point to come back to.

Hearing information with others can be very validating, and having some idea of how people live, manage and heal can offer hope and a sense of solidarity. Groups for people with the same condition can be very supportive, although not universally so.

Table 3.1 gives examples of initial work clinicians can engage in depending on the resources available. This will include financial and social support as well as information about the condition and establishing self-management goals. Peer support can be used to facilitate elements of this.

Table 3.1 Case examples

Example	Initial plan
Steve is a builder who also regularly cycled competitively in long distance races. He lives with his partner. He contracted Covid-19 a year ago, and has been seen by respiratory and cardiac clinics and no pathology was found; he remains significantly fatigued and experiences aches and pain. His cognitive function is affected with challenges in concentration, attention and word finding. He is signed off work. He has been suicidal and has been in touch with the crisis team.	Confirming the Long Covid diagnosis, signposting him for financial help and reports to support his welfare benefits application; introducing Steve to others living with Long Covid, learning about the condition and starting to set self-management goals, for example around sleep, and working with him to start very small amounts of physical activity rather than pushing to do a lot or doing nothing. Maintaining contact and monitoring his emotional health.

Aysha was an active director of a company who enjoyed long walks at the weekends and socialized with friends. She lives alone. She contracted a viral infection after losing her mum to a long-term illness two years ago. She feels she has never fully recovered, is working part-time from home, socializes rarely. Only goes out if she must. Has had extensive investigations.	Information about the condition that fulfils criteria for ME/CFS; review with her what seems important to her – which she identified as seeing friends and going out more – and work out with her ways she could start this. A series of appointments to review understanding and changes she is making; consider a facilitated group to gain support from peers.
Jenny is a teacher diagnosed with fibromyalgia; she is not sure how she developed it but experiences pervasive pain that at times affects her mobility and mental processing, including word finding and concentration. She is applying for early retirement from teaching as she found her cognitive attention and her mobility and balance meant she was not consistently able to manage a class even with a reduction in hours, specialized seating and additional teaching assistant help.	Detailed functional report and occupational history to support retirement. Looking at how she has managed so far, providing ways of learning about the condition and setting goals and priorities going forward.

Clinician's use of mindfulness at this stage

While it is not directly 'mindfulness', an intrinsic part of the mindfulness-based approach is to have carefully identified what the problem is. Furthermore, mindfulness can support how the client and the clinician work together to find a way to look at the challenges. The clinician's use of mindfulness to regulate themselves, to really listen and give space to the person who is living through a very knotty situation, can lean into their own practice (Pollak et al. 2014). The therapeutic use of self is well documented; without an easy answer or technology to manage these problems, we have to use our own experience and approach. People will have been trying for months, for years, to address their problems and may have paid for help too. Acknowledging all of this and the fact that if it was easy they would not be here is important. Not immediately jumping in to problem-solving or advice-giving, but rather hearing and validating someone's experience, can help the individual find a way forward and consider how the service can help (Chew-Graham et al. 2011).

SUMMARY

- While ME/CFS, fibromyalgia and Long Covid are distinct conditions that warrant specific diagnosis and treatment options, there are similarities in both symptoms and experience to generate a transdiagnostic rehabilitative approach, and a model of dysregulated system seems to describe people's experience with these health conditions. There are no confirmatory tests for these conditions, so diagnosis is made through description of symptoms, their history and impact.
- The symptoms have a post-exertional nature which can result in 'boom and bust' in activity, which means a prolonged period of recovery can be required following participation in activity. This can be hard to manage, understand or explain.
- Support needs to consider what medical management may be possible (e.g. pain, sleep, mood medication) and the practical, social, employment, financial and psychological impact of the symptoms.
- The individual with the condition needs to have appropriate information and set their own priorities for treatment/intervention.

Chapter 4

Supported Self-Management

- Summary of self-management
- Difficulties that can arise for patients and clinicians
- The challenges a mindfulness-based approach can support

We normally go to a hospital appointment expecting to see a doctor who can offer us some treatment or cure, often in the form of medicine or surgery. The 'treatment' for fatigue and persistent pain is often guided self-management, which has a physiological basis but is entirely implemented by the patient. Supported self-management is a whole process and book in itself. Coakley and Knops's *Living with ME and Chronic Fatigue Syndrome* (2022) is particularly clear on what this involves. Action for ME and the ME Association also have detailed information on their websites (see the Resources section).

The main principles of supported self-management include the following:

- Coming to an understanding of the physical, mental, social and emotional factors and identifying that medication and time alone are not enough
- Agreeing that lifestyle changes are likely to help and specific strategies for different circumstances can be developed
- Establishing a balance of sleep, rest, meals, movement, and must-do and enjoyable activity
- Working out personal levels of high, medium and low activity
- Learning how to rest
- Establishing baseline (or sustainable) levels of activity to balance out unsustainable boom-and-bust pattern of activity. Baselines can be physical, cognitive or emotional.
- Setting goals or a focus in life
- Prioritizing activity over a day, a week, a month (which conversely means de-prioritizing some activity and perhaps significantly changing personal standards)
- Pacing or spreading out activity.

APPLYING THE PRINCIPLES OF SUPPORTED SELF-MANAGEMENT

Baselines

Samir works out he can walk for ten minutes a day and still manage other tasks; if he walks for half an hour, he cannot walk or do much else for three or four days afterwards, which is a net reduction compared to a ten-minute daily walk plus other daily tasks.

Julie was regularly managing three to four hours of activity a day, but had some stress in her communication with her employer which reduced her activity to two to three hours (because the communication and stress used up more energy). Noticing that her baseline was a 'lower' number of hours but of higher intensity helped her manage both practically and emotionally.

Setting goals or a focus in life

Samir's focus is on spending time with his children – so he prioritizes activities with them over other activity such as seeing friends or gardening, which he still does but moderates and plans them.

Prioritizing activity

Julie's focus is on work and her finances but knows she does need to see friends and family to feel better, so balances this over a month and uses her annual leave strategically.

Pacing activity

Because Samir wants to prioritize his family, he does some work at home in the morning, then rests from lunchtime until 2:30pm with a combination of relaxation techniques and light activity (e.g. listening to the radio or sitting in his garden) so he can have dinner with his children, be involved with the evening routine and also spend some time with his partner.

Supported self-management has several phases:

1. *Defining the situation/problem.* Therapist and patient agree together not only that the diagnosis fits but that the understanding of the condition fits their experience. Can they place their symptoms, the history of their symptoms

and their experience of their symptoms into the framework suggested by the alarm-system model? And do they want to work within this?

2. *Education* – not only about the condition but also about ways that the model can be applied and turned into actionable changes that increase a sense of control and engagement in meaningful activity to improve function and quality of life.

3. *Development of an individualized plan* to include what will be worked on and how this needs supporting; for example, changes to sleep patterns supported by using a diary, checking in with a therapist every month, and referral to a group programme to support implementation of baselined activity management.

4. *Addressing particular challenges* within a multi-disciplinary team or providing consultancy to other teams; for example, digestive problems, sleep problems, pain in particular areas, physical weakness, employment issues, family and social issues, financial problems, anxiety, past trauma. These need to be addressed within the context of managing a fluctuating health condition and the need for a paced approach. These challenges mean it is helpful to have a multi-disciplinary team of physiotherapists, occupational therapists, psychologists and dieticians as well as access to specialists in sleep and pain management and to be aware of local services, such as employment advisers, housing specialists, and trauma and mental health services.

5. *Reviews* initially scheduled and then on request as patient initiated follow-ups.

Difficulties with self-management

Everyone has a unique genetic and social makeup and past that means we are all likely to interpret the same event in our own particular way. Services need to be able to individualize the approach according to each person. For some, baselining activity, learning to rest effectively, exercise at an appropriate and manageable level, stabilizing sleep, and so on, can lead to a full recovery. In the case of post-viral fatigue, there will be a natural recovery that can be optimized by meaningful management. Some with a more chronic presentation may *feel* better, but are not better. In others, the condition can last for several years, over which time there would have been changes anyway, we just don't know what they would have been (Cheshire et al. 2021).

We are unable to be clear about how long someone will be unwell; this is particularly pronounced in situations when others have the same precipitating illness, such as Covid-19, which others may have had at the same time and are now completely better (we are seeing people who have had Long Covid at disabling levels now for over three years). This lack of certainty about how long the situation will go on for understandably adds to the confusion and fear: 'Do I make permanent arrangements regarding my work? Is it better to rest up completely to give myself a chance of recovery?' Then there may be days or even weeks when things pick up: 'I had three days last week when I felt normal', which can be exciting, but can also lead to doubts about what is going on – 'Am I really ill? Am I doing this to myself?' This can lead to bigger questions around identity and who one is, particularly if the idea of 'self' is conflated with 'what I do'.

As well as the symptoms being difficult, the nature of the conditions means there are challenges in:

- the process of coming to a diagnosis
- recovering from an initial illness but remaining unwell (many people have been extremely unwell with an acute health condition and this of itself is traumatic)
- the fluctuating (often 'boom-and-bust') nature of the symptoms, which means working out what one can do is both complicated and time-consuming
- the status of the condition and external beliefs and attitudes in the world (this is not real illness; people with ME/CFS, fibromyalgia or Long Covid are attention-seeking, lazy freeloaders)
- internal beliefs such as 'my condition is not real', 'if I rest I'm being lazy; people think I'm shirking'; some people say that they didn't previously believe that ME/CFS or fibromyalgia, etc. were real and that they weren't the 'kind of people' to get that kind of illness.

More than coping?

Self-management sounds like it's about coping, but if we consider the theory of dysregulation outlined in the previous chapter, that posits the body's processes are fluctuating between exertion and collapse in response to an overactive protective system. It follows that stabilizing physiological routines such as sleep, mealtimes and how much the body moves may lead to more balance and regulation. Learning to 'down-regulate' through effective rest, planning and pacing encourages a more gentle flip-flop between being active and resting (going between the sympathetic and parasympathetic systems or up-regulating and down-regulating over the day), creating the potential to make things better.

However, doing this in order to 'fix things' adds a pressure that counteracts this intention, and if it doesn't work can 'worry' the system so the 'protective mode' is agitated again. The somewhat paradoxical challenge is to carry out the changes in a way that serves what we care about, and enables life to be lived now, rather than with the goal of getting better or being a particular type of person.

And perhaps the worst that can happen with a skilful management approach is that someone can live in a way that is meaningful and satisfying for them right now. This of itself is the basis of recovery.

In many ways the specialism in this field is not the technique but the capacity to sit with a person, hear what is going on, help them construct a valid narrative about what happened and develop a way forward with support for the sticky areas.

How clinicians support these challenges

There is quite a lot to accept and this can be addressed by the clinician in both implicit and explicit ways. The work that has been done on trauma-informed practice offers a system that could be applied here – the 5 Rs offer a useful summary: Realize; Recognize; Respond; Resist retraumatizing: and Referral (Gold in Crane et al. 2021).

- *Realize* the multifactorial nature of the situation is challenging.
- *Recognize* distress, grief, unacceptance and that there is a lot to 'accept'. This is complex.
- *Respond* with care, belief and acknowledgement of struggle with the process of self-management as much as with the symptoms.
- *Resist retraumatizing* by disbelieving or by sending them on another hunt for more tests (if you have clarified that adequate tests have been done, e.g. see NICE guidance) or another 'cure', not being able to offer any support.
- *Referral* (if appropriate) to another team (e.g. mental health team for depression, PTSD; social services, financial advice; employment services, etc.) or to a colleague with a different skill set or more experience.

SUMMARY

- Supported self-management requires a clear assessment of the individual's situation.
- As it is 'self-management', the patient needs to have information and understanding about the condition and what may help.
- There needs to be access to a range of professionals including different medical specialties as well as a range of clinicians who can refer to other sectors such as housing and mental health services.
- While this approach does not address the mechanisms of the illness, physiological stabilization can support people feeling somewhat better.

- The approach needs to have the individual at the heart of the process and provide support in working through challenges including financial and social problems.
- Clinicians need support and supervision and good team networks to support this approach.

Chapter 5

What Is a Mindfulness-Based Approach?

- Definitions of mindfulness
- An approach to difficulty
- Reactions to difficulties and seeing that things change
- Identity and sense of self

Defining mindfulness

Mindfulness has become a ubiquitous term for many things, from a synonym for being calm or peaceful and taking a moment, to a marketing tool for herbal teabags, notebooks, colouring books, walks, yoga classes and the type of clothes and food we buy. It is an important part of Buddhist psychology and practice and there are numerous teachings and discourses on mindfulness and its role in practices that have the relief of suffering at their core. I struggle to define it even though I have an MSc in mindfulness-based approaches, am sitting in a room full of books on the subject and have folder after folder of articles on my computer. It has been part of my life for several decades and is in my job title, 'Mindfulness Based Therapist' (Bishop 2004; van Dam et al. 2018).

It seems definitions abound; while there are pages and pages devoted to the subject, I repeatedly return to two places:

- Jon Kabat-Zinn's (2013) definition: 'Mindfulness is awareness that arises through paying attention, on purpose, in the present moment, non-judgementally.' To which he added in an article in 2017: 'in the service of self-understanding and wisdom'.
- Shapiro's description of the mechanisms of mindfulness place that definition into a model that informs the practice, application and the way mindfulness is taught (Crane et al. 2021; Shapiro et al. 2006). This model describes the processes in all mindfulness practices, whether they are

formal meditation-based practices or informal daily activity. It breaks Kabat-Zinn's definition of mindfulness into three axioms (Figure 5.1):

- *Intention*: What do we mean to do? That is, which practice or activity; doing what we are doing on purpose.
- *Attitude*: How one practises and the attitudes to the practice or activity are fundamental. Kabat-Zinn called these attitudes 'the attitudinal foundations of mindfulness'. They are: non-judging, patience, acceptance, non-striving, trust, letting go and beginner's mind (Kabat-Zinn 2013).
- *Attention*: Where are we placing our attention? Body, breath, sounds, thoughts. Or within the components of an activity, e.g. stirring porridge; washing up a dish; walking our child to school. Can we place our attention, even if it is just for a few moments, on what we are actually doing?

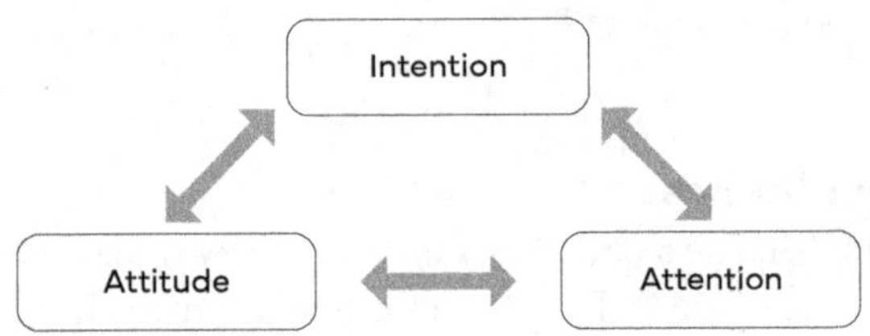

Figure 5.1 Three axioms of mindfulness (Shapiro et al. 2006)

The three axioms work together and influence what is attended to and how the attending happens. This can lead to a 'decentred' awareness that enables one to step back and 'reperceive' the moment, but can also lead to a fundamental shift in understanding that may change how other aspects of life are approached. This is the way mindfulness enables insight and wisdom that supports the creation of a more fulfilling life. The approach is based in contemporary cognitive science and current understanding of how humans function as well as in contemplative wisdom, particularly Buddhism, that has addressed the challenge of life for millennia.

Jon Kabat-Zinn's seminal work on mindfulness-based stress reduction (MBSR) took the Buddhist philosophy, psychology and approach and:

> recontextualise[d] it within the frameworks of science, medicine (including psychiatry and psychology), and healthcare so that it would be maximally useful to people who could not hear it or enter into it through the more traditional dharma gates, whether they were doctors or medical patients. (Kabat-Zinn 2013)

Meanwhile, mindfulness-based cognitive therapy (MBCT) (Segal et al. 2013) developed from the other direction. Researchers found that recurrent depression could be treated with an approach that was very similar to contemplative methods and the MBSR programme was incorporated into this form of cognitive therapy to become MBCT. Cognitive science and contemporary contemplative practice have continued to work together and inform the development of mindfulness-based approaches, and contemporary imaging studies and neuroscience have added to the field.

Understanding difficulty

Mindfulness-based programmes at their heart address the human question of how we can live a good life when life is so difficult. In health settings mindfulness-based programmes support people with a specific challenge: How can I live with an unwanted health condition?

In order to make the approach applicable to our daily lives, the approach is practice-based and experiential; in other words, one does not have to understand the theory, just do the practice: '...we are never appealing to authority or tradition, only to the richness of the present moment held gently in awareness, and the profound and authentic authority of each person's own experience, equally held with kindness in awareness' (Kabat-Zinn 2013).

Kabat-Zinn's packaging is deceptively simple, so much is covered within the MBSR programme. When we bring awareness to our lives, one often notices things are frequently not how we want them to be. Understanding the nature of the problem is a key first step and this is looked at next.

The basic mechanism of our struggle with difficulty and the path through it is based on four factors (known as the Four Noble Truths in Buddhism) and reconceptualized as four tasks by Stephen Batchelor (2017) and also described by the Breathworks programme (Burch and Penman 2013). An adapted version of these four factors for managing fatigue syndromes is offered here:

1. Life has challenges and we struggle and suffer; there are problems in life and some of them are not easily remedied and have further consequences (e.g. a fatiguing health condition that seems to have no easy medical answer and reduces our capacity to work or even take care of ourselves), so we struggle.

2. None of us like having problems that have no obvious answer, so we frequently react by having a problem with the problem, and either ignore it (and hope it will go away) or fight it, but this fight doesn't solve the problem. Both reactions – ignoring or fighting – mean the problem can create additional problems and we feel even worse.

3. It is possible to stop habitually fighting or ignoring the problem and,

even if we can't stop the initial problem, we can address the consequences. We can have more control and feel better. In other words, we can respond and find some peace.

4. We can learn skills to manage our difficulties. There are ways to do this that have been tried out by others and we can learn how to do this and have some support.

Each point links: By seeing that I have a problem with the problem, I am already starting to see what can be done. By stopping the problem with the problem, I am already reducing the problem. By considering what can be done, I can see a way to how this can happen. By understanding what happens, I can change and perhaps prevent the situation getting worse, and there may be a way through this I currently do not know.

It may sound simple, but humans are complex, and some problems are knotty, we may need some help, and that's where therapists and others come in. Additionally, the fundamental root of many problems cannot be eradicated, either because they are insurmountable or because they happened in the past and have irrevocably led to the current situation. This could be an injury, a war, child abuse or contracting a virus. It has happened, and we are left living with the consequences. How these consequences express themselves in an individual is unique due to their cultural, genetic and individual histories as well as their current social, economic and cultural context. Therapy and related fields (such as spiritual practices) have developed ways to support people, first by looking at the problem with all its layers and consequences (which can of itself change how we relate and reduce some of the suffering); and secondly by considering what can be done, bearing in mind our understanding now.

First and second arrows

A version of the Buddhist story of the arrows describes the first two factors and how this may look. The story of the arrows is a shortcut way to think about difficulty and how we respond to it (Figure 5.2). The first arrow represents the 'pain of pain', the reality of what has happened. The second arrow is our reaction to what has happened, what we add to the experience through avoiding, struggling and pushing away. This second arrow creates more suffering and compounds the problems.

For example, Sasha had Covid, was in hospital, came out, seemed to be recovering and went back to work but was not able to manage more than two days before going off sick. She is referred to the clinic a year later having lost her job and become socially isolated with deteriorating mental health. This is unarguably hard, distressing and difficult on a day-to-day basis.

The first arrow represents the problem: She had Covid, was very ill and, despite trying and wanting to, was not able to work and struggled to see her friends and family. There is no obvious cure for Long Covid, and the pattern of fluctuating symptoms can be hard to manage.

The second arrow represents her reactions: She kept going, not telling anyone, and experienced significant post-exertional symptoms that she hid from everyone, resulting in her not seeing people at all. She became increasingly isolated and her mood lowered. She continued not being able to work and eventually lost her job and couldn't face looking into benefits or other support, so used up all her savings to live. She now had physical health problems, financial and housing difficulties and her mental health was affected as well as having Long Covid.

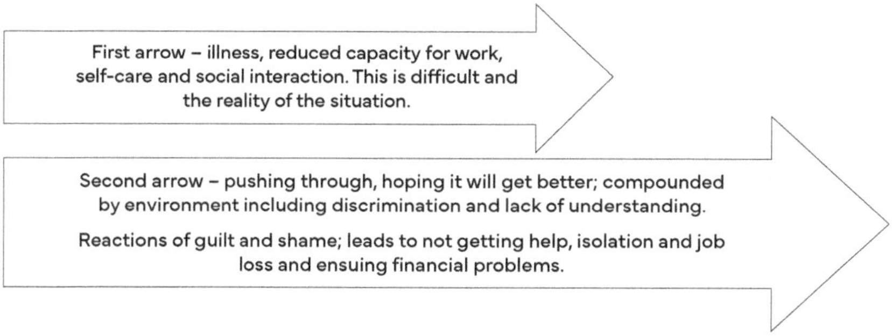

Figure 5.2 The two arrows

There are many reasons why people end up in this situation; in her case Sasha may not have had any advice or help when she left hospital. Her GP may not have appreciated that she was going off work and had no means of financial support and a vulnerable work situation. Others had Covid at the time and are now recovered, so why isn't she? She may have a longstanding pattern of keeping going regardless; she may have had an unsupportive workplace. The pandemic created huge uncertainty and change particularly in some sectors. It will be different for each person. Looking at the facts of the situation, the reality of Long Covid, job loss, isolation and financial hardship is painful. The impact of the symptoms means it can be difficult to address the problem, and confusion and shame about what the symptoms are compounds the problem.

Being able to address this spiralling situation with medical, mental health, employment and housing challenges is hard, and having someone alongside may be the only way to make this possible.

We were able to support Sasha by initially laying out the problem and worked with her to ascertain what she needed to do about the second arrow, and broke it down into manageable amounts. First, we looked at finance and benefits and arranged to call her once a week for 15 minutes to look at where she was and what she had managed to sort out and then problem-solve with her. Then, using a process we developed with her, we helped her make a plan, so that she realistically planned and paced the next step. Within eight weeks she got the hang of the approach, had various things in place and was setting up support with benefit applications and debt management and was back in touch with some friends who helped her with the house. She then felt able to join a Long Covid self-management group for some support with going forward.

While this may not look like a mindfulness-based approach (where is the meditation?), it is, however, the four-stage process in action: the conversations with healthcare practitioners (from the GP to the assessing therapist in the Long Covid clinic) helped her to identify what was going on and notice the patterns of reactivity (in this case overwhelm and withdrawal). While there is no obvious medical answer, she was able to look in detail at what had happened and practical steps were identified to start to address the secondary problems. From this there was an opportunity to go on to address symptoms and ways of managing day-to-day life that may lead her to better health. Seeing the reality in a complete way, including problems caused by social exclusion and inequality, will affect how help is offered.

The self-management approach keeps the individual in charge and making choices. Another person who was not able to access the help in the way Sasha did, because they were so unwell and needed help with self-care for example, would need help in accessing social care. This means having a service that is aware of where this help lies, and access to advocates and other agencies is a part of the approach and the challenge of working in this way.

Because there is no easy medical answer, it can feel overwhelming, and individuals can feel they are to blame and somehow responsible for it all. Navigating this alongside the person with the health condition is a crucial skill for practitioners as it gives glimpses of the third and fourth 'truths' – experiencing a way to respond to the situation and that there seems to be a way through some of the knots. Understanding 'I am not the only one who feels like this and that others feel this too' (evidenced by the fact that there are services that help) is a key part of learning to respond. Questions that can be asked by both the person with the health problem and the healthcare practitioner include:

- 'What is the reality of this situation? What are the facts?'
- 'How can I take care of myself within this situation? What could help?'

However, the context and tone of these questions is important if one is going to be able to first see the situation and then take steps to change. In other words, insight must first be cultivated and then choices can be made, and plans put in place based on understanding and choice (as opposed to fear and reaction).

Creating the conditions for insight

The Merriam-Webster online dictionary defines insight as:

1. the power or act of seeing into a situation: penetration
2. the act or result of apprehending the inner nature of things or of seeing intuitively.

In both Buddhism and contemporary cognitive science, it is recognized that in order to get to a point where one can gain insight and make changes that alleviate suffering, one needs to create the conditions whereby insight can arise. Gilbert and Choden (2013) use the Tibetan Buddhist meanings of meditation: *familiarization* and *cultivation* – that is, we familiarize ourselves with our reactive minds and tendencies and the ways this leads us into particular ways of think-ing and acting. We can also observe what helps us, what is more 'wholesome', kind and useful to ourselves and others, and cultivate and develop these ways of being. In order to do this, a more open and responsive mind state needs to be accessible, which means both feeling safe and feeling calm (Gilbert 2020). Therefore, some background work may need to be completed before insight is developed, and we can 'do' what looks like a mindfulness approach where we sit in a circle and meditate.

Creating the environment for mindfulness: Stabilization

When one is living with a complex array of problems including the health and social problems that can come when living with a complex condition, it can be challenging to see what is going on. It can feel like living in a never-ending and ever-tightening knot, so 'stabilizing' can be challenging (Gilbert 2020; Gilbert and Choden 2013). Shame and isolation are particularly strong features, and in the above example of Sasha we can see how that plays out as she was not able to ask for help until her life had become extremely difficult and her basic needs were threatened. In considering this, we need to go beyond the individual and beyond the individual therapist who may be working with people like Sasha and consider the wider picture and how we as therapists/helpers interact with the wider context (Figure 5.3).

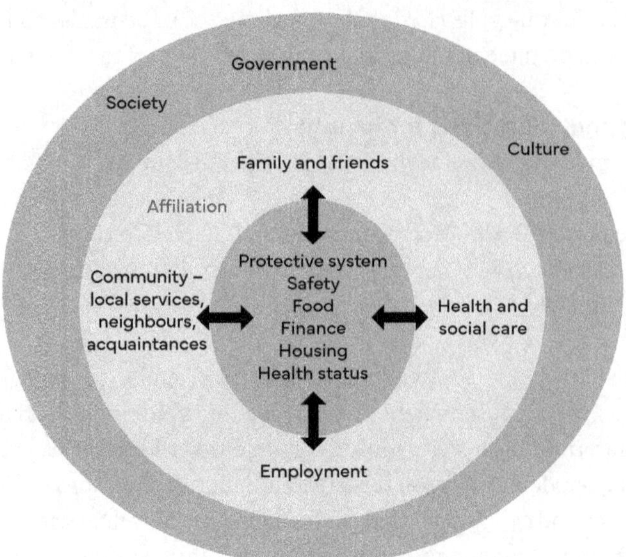

Figure 5.3 The wider context

Humans (and other animals) have a primal protection system that keeps them safe from predators as well as ensuring access to shelter, food and reproduction. In order to survive, there is a need for affiliation and connection to a social group. In Sasha's example she survived on her own for so long, then needed to have some help, from health services, advice agencies and from her friends. In modern societies, things are complicated as we need to work and have formalized some of our systems into health and social care. This requires social organization on cultural and governmental levels, perhaps outside of our sphere of influence. Sasha's example shows that to receive help, one must be able to ask for help. But this can be difficult if there is lack of knowledge in the system about what to do or cultural 'disbelief' in particular conditions; for example, some people with ME meet disbelief from health professionals as well as employers, family and friends, and it may not be possible to ask for help as there is no service in the area.

In a service that does exist, if health professionals do not see their role as offering support in accessing help with (or at least information about) employment and financial concerns, this affects the capacity of the person with the health condition as they are in survival mode, frightened (Pilkington et al. 2020) and unable to access the approach that is offered. It can take time for the individual to feel safe enough to tell someone about their situation and the impact it has. If a service is very limited in personnel or hours each patient can have, then there may not be enough safety in the system for some. This is exacerbated if someone is from a marginalized group through class, race, poverty, language, education, nationality, sex, gender, sexual orientation, and so on. Part of accessing help is having the confidence and ability to spot that this problem is something that can be helped and there are people and services to help.

Stabilization, therefore, starts long before we formally teach people mindfulness. The first conversations with someone who understands and cares and a collaborative plan is emerging can really help. Mindfulness practice in those early stages can help people access some comfort and calm through feeling the contact with the floor, feeling of their body on the chair, the flow of breath and perhaps access a comforting image or memory. Both patients and clinicians need to be aware of the potential to be overwhelmed by the magnitude of the situation and make achievable and actionable goals to start. As we will see, ensuring the person with the health condition has control and the process is centred on their whole experience is important.

The nature of distress

Understanding the nature of why we may respond to a problem can help, and the following principles from Buddhism that underpin the implicit curriculum of mindfulness-based courses point to ways of managing suffering and distress (Crane 2017b).

- We react because life is full of things we don't like.
- Everything changes, but appreciating this is difficult and causes us distress.
- Our identity is not fixed. 'I' is the result of a number of variables. Not seeing this also adds to our distress and sometimes we need to grieve for who we feel we once were. However, seeing that we have different roles and identities can be freeing.

Reaction

All living beings automatically react with aversion to a noxious stimulus by moving away. It is how living things stay alive. We pull away from things that are very hot, that will pierce our outer physical layer (skin, fur, feathers, scales). We have sensors that detect problems and complex reactions that enable us to get away: the nerve sensors in eyes, ears and skin detect a problem; the endocrine system secretes hormones that stimulate us to move fast; the heart and lungs pump faster to enable the system to be fuelled; the immediate response of muscles that coordinate on order to enable us to be safe, and so on. It is automatic and quite miraculous; we don't need to think it through.

This is OK when this solves the problem. The problem arises when it doesn't, when the problem stays or is not fixed no matter how fast we run. In the animal world, we can see this as freeze or playing dead until the danger passes (think of a cat playing with a mouse, the mouse will freeze and appear dead and the cat gets bored as it is no longer moving).

In health conditions that don't have easy answers, this reaction can be exhausting of itself, and we can end up endlessly pursuing treatments that at best do nothing, and find it hard to keep steady or cope with the basics of life. As we have seen, sometimes the priority needs to be managing finances and housing rather than fruitlessly searching for something to get us better so we can return to how life was.

Identifying when we are unhelpfully reacting or when the reaction is not going to change anything and when a considered, perhaps very different, response is required is key (Figure 5.4).

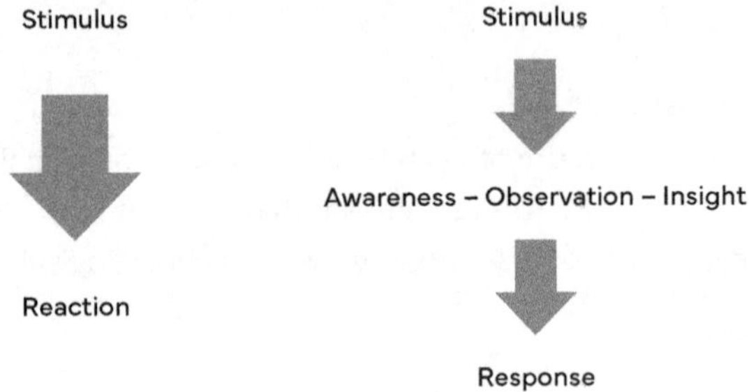

Figure 5.4 Reacting vs. responding

Mindfulness puts in a pause between the stimulus and reaction; this may be immediately obvious, we notice we are scared and flinch when a large dog barks at us in the park. That is obvious; sometimes the stimulus/reaction is more complex, as in the example of Paul (see box).

PAUL

Paul found himself cleaning the whole flat, again. He realized again he had 'just' done this *again* despite the impact he was starting to feel in his back and limbs. From past experience he knew that he could expect this to progress for the next day or so and he would have debilitating fatigue, feeling like he had flu, nausea, and so on, and that this would mean he would need to cancel tomorrow night's date with his boyfriend Tim. Again.

Paul's immediate reaction was to feel angry at himself and his illness; he also had the thought he might have got away with it, so would carry on regardless and see if he could manage the date, and then found himself weighing up different excuses he could make to cancel... He was feeling tense, frustrated and upset.

Paul was learning mindfulness, so he decided to take a break, sit down, and listen to a body scan. The half hour of gently moving through the body, breathing gently and 'as best he could' unravelling any tension that could be eased. His thinking slowed down and by the end he drifted off and felt relaxed. He recalled the expression to consider a response instead of reacting and wondered what this might mean. If he responded by resting now and didn't do some of the other jobs he was meant to today, despite feeling relatively OK and they needed doing… If instead he rested, listened to an audio book and walked to a local shop, he could get some simple things to cook for Tim instead of going out to the pub and for a meal… If he didn't feel well enough to cook, he could get a takeaway… He also considered that perhaps it was time he explained to Tim about his health and not just see him when he was OK or cancel with some made-up reason.

Paul considered this and noticed that, by pausing and reflecting, things were changing already. He texted Tim, told him he wasn't feeling like the pub and asked what he would prefer. Tim it turns out was relieved, he had started to get used to Paul bailing out of their dates and was worried that the text was another cancellation and what that might mean. He offered to bring some food and they could cook together. Paul then noticed that he had gone from tense, fatigued and anxious to relaxed, cheerful and hopeful. He then chose to rest with his audio book.

Paul's situation is an example of moving from reaction to a situation to finding a way to reflect and consider options. He had been locked in a cycle of pushing through, and only seeing Tim at the times when he was OK. Spotting that perhaps this was getting in the way of what he cared about and starting to cause problems (not only with Tim, but with other friends and family) meant that he could start to see if there were other ways. It also gave rise to another observation: everything changes.

Everything changes

We cannot control most things – we cannot control the weather, the traffic, what is happening on the other side of the world, or even next door. And no matter how wonderful or sad something is, it will always change: the beautiful sun will set; the party will end; the sea will come in; the grass will grow; we stop crying. Mindfulness offers a way to see the change, to notice our feelings arise and fall, much like the weather. With the ability to respond, we can tend to this moment. We may start with occasional glimpses of responding like this; even if we have intellectually understood impermanence, living it is another matter.

Spotting that we feel it is fixed and hopeless and that there is no way out and that is frightening may well be all we can do. A question that can perhaps help is: 'What's the weather today?' And, again, we can ask: 'How can I take care of myself?'

A sense of fixed identity

There can be problems if we have fixed ideas about what makes us the people we are: 'I am a tidy person', 'I am determined', 'I am spontaneous' – these qualities may well be a predominant part of character and behaviour and are important, but seeing these traits as immutable elements of oneself can lead to additional struggle and pain when faced with a health condition that prevents their being realized:

- 'Who am I if I don't work in a job that involves international travel and don't run ultra-marathons in my spare time?'
- 'Who am I if I cannot pick my kids up from school and play on the beach?'

In both these cases, there is grief for who they were, fear of the future and huge uncertainty at how life is run. The first example may sound like a more privileged loss, but the void at not being able to work as one always has (and the risk of losing a livelihood that has been built up) and loss of entire social life can be excruciating. Even more so if the other aspects of ourselves are not only not in view or recognized but are dismissed as lesser ways of being – 'perhaps OK for others but that's not me'; therefore the struggle becomes existential anguish: 'Who am I?' and 'What is important?'

Mindfulness practices cultivate a way of being with ourself initially by 'watching' thoughts, sounds, sensations as they arise and change, as though we were watching a film or sitting on a river bank. This process enables us to see that:

- we like some things, and don't like or are indifferent to others
- things do change
- there is a part of us that can observe all of this, so perhaps our idea that we are a fixed personality with absolute thoughts is not actually true.

This understanding can lead to an inquiry as to 'who is the observer?', but this could become very complicated, so keep the practice grounded in what is here and now: the experience of the moment in an embodied way by inhabiting each moment, as opposed to what we *think* about each moment, enables the recognition that things change and that we are literally not who we 'think' we are (Nairn, Choden and Regan-Addis 2019).

ANDREI

Andrei was an active dad to two girls, and loved taking them cycling, swimming and playing on the trampoline. He was a successful triathlete and ran his own business. After contracting dengue fever on a work trip abroad, then catching Covid six months later, he had significant symptoms and was affected in all aspects of daily life, struggling to walk, concentrate and socialize even within his family. While he understood and managed to delegate his work and gave up his sports, his identity as a dad was a struggle. He felt a huge sense of loss at not being able to be the active dad he previously was. This resulted in him withdrawing, which affected his relationships with his partner as well as his daughters.

Part of his therapy included looking at what was important to him and how he could manage this: by focusing on what he could do and translating that into activities he could do with his children. With careful planning and pacing he was now able to occasionally drive and walk short distances and started being able to meet the girls and his partner at the end of their bike rides and tracked their progress through mobile phone GPS. He made them picnics for the end and helped them work out routes and maintain their bikes. His identity as a dad was important, but how it was enacted changed; managing his grief for the loss of his important role and finding ways to inhabit this aspect of himself meant he could find a way through and maintain closeness with his children. He reflected and said that he would have had to find new ways at some point as the girls grew up or if their interests changed.

His partner was relieved to have an active co-parent again and felt it was a good indicator that while he was not 'who he was' physically, he was back to being the person she knew and they could work together to maintain family life.

SUMMARY

- Mindfulness definitions abound; we are using Jon Kabat-Zinn's definition: 'Mindfulness is awareness that arises through paying attention, on purpose, in the present moment, non-judgementally.'
- Shapiro's axioms of mindfulness describe how daily activity as well as formal practices can be mindful by considering intention, attention and attitude.
- Mindfulness-based programmes at their heart address the human question of how we can live a good life when life is so difficult. In health

settings mindfulness-based programmes support people with a specific challenge: How can I live with an unwanted health condition?

- Understanding the nature of the challenge and the problems caused by avoidance and overwhelm are key to finding a way forward.
- Understanding, compassion and non-judgement are important to finding a way forward and are cultivated within the therapist as well as within the person with the health condition.

Chapter 6

Mindfulness-Based Approach to Self-Management

- A summary of how mindfulness can support self-management
- Acceptance of the current situation can help individuals address where they are in a constructive way that supports a way forward
- A mindfulness-based approach can complement and enhance self-management strategies such as sleep management, pacing and resting

As we have seen, the process of clarifying the problem, the clinician's stance of curious non-judgemental interest, giving time to understanding, and the person with the health condition going at a pace that supports them making considered responses to the information, is all good clinical practice that can be supported by a mindfulness-based approach. Directly teaching and learning mindfulness could support self-management in the following ways:

- Mindfulness practices, while not necessarily relaxing, can support regulation and can enhance sleep, rest, digestion and pain management. Our programme emphasizes the 'down-regulating' and the relaxation response as a basis and resource building for each person.
- Observing patterns of behaviour and the role of thoughts can be useful. The invitation to practise at home can show up challenges in finding ways to manage; these can be practical hurdles or social or emotional difficulties.
- The development of practices that use the body and the moment we are in to guide us serves the current situation better than relying entirely on habitual thoughts and behaviour patterns.

Clearly, this is not simple, and as we have discussed, the context for doing this is involved. Mindfulness-based programmes offer a way to hold all of this by:

- using the practices with specific intentions (calming, understanding, choices)

- setting aside time for practice
- teaching mindfulness practices over the weeks with increasing complexity, knowing that it is possible to come back to just the moment and pause and take care and that any action taken is from a place of gently settling and pausing
- inquiring into experience and a shared experience with others in similar situations support both the learning of mindfulness and application to daily life.

Acceptance of a change changes everything, but also *doesn't* change everything (children still need to be cared for, houses cleaned, finance managed). It is how we go about tasks that is transformed and very different. For people who are severely affected, these tasks may need to be taken on completely by others as even getting to the toilet is difficult and conversations may be limited to minutes at a time.

Alongside adapting to the condition and making changes there is understandable resentment, sadness, grief, anger and confusion. There is also sometimes joy, relief and excitement and the potential to have new experiences that perhaps we were not open to (or even aware of). Mindfulness enables individuals to see things how they are now while taking care of how they feel about the situation.

The attention to moment-by-moment awareness and experience and the constant flux of change means there is a potential to notice when things are easier, changing and improving as much as they are challenging. By focusing on this moment, both what is going on and what is needed can make this moment manageable and start to create a series of linked moments. These small changes can add up, as the examples of Jenny, Nikolaus and Nina show (see box).

JENNY

Jenny caught Covid-19 and 18 months later was continuing to struggle to manage daily life; she needed help with cooking and housework and could only manage short walks. She was worried about breathlessness and what that meant. She knew that her lungs were not damaged but was unclear how to progress. Learning to come to the body, relax her shoulders and gently breathe felt better and her breathing became easier. She could do a little more and gradually was able to do more by pacing out her activity and slowing down her movements and her breath. Jenny also noticed the link with feeling stressed (e.g. dealing with her finances), when she became fatigued, struggled to walk and her breathing became laboured. She practised awareness of her reactions and also noticed that lowering her shoulders and gently breathing eased some of her tension and fatigue and cleared space to think. She described the feeling of control over her body:

> I can do something, my body feels easier, and when I do this, I can find alternative ways to look at things. I also remember other times that I have coped (e.g. being made redundant). I can ask questions and seek help rather than waiting for it all to come at me and then tumble down out of control. I also realize that my imagination is often worse than reality, and the reality is I often need more information to sort things out. If I don't ask, I won't know what to do. If I know what to do, I can find a way to do something about it even if it is tiny steps.

NIKOLAUS

Nikolaus, a hospital medic (post-glandular fever), noted that if he took short breaks and pauses and used the mindfulness pause and check-in with what his priorities were and then how he needed to progress into the next moment, he could focus and concentrate better and reported less exhaustion at the end of his shift and was able to sleep better.

NINA

Nina worked in retail and during her extended phased return with Long Covid she negotiated being able to sit at her job and found that if she did a half-hour practice on returning home (as well as short check-ins throughout the day), she had fewer symptoms and was able to spend some time with her family in the evenings. She also found that her digestion improved.

As well as learning to 'down-regulate', the mindfulness-based programme includes:

- regular practices that support the development and enhancement of routines that are individualized and based on the individual's lifestyle
- movement practices that encourage and support curiosity and compassion, moving in a way that the body can now, with an awareness of 'pushing' or extending that may be appropriate, but may be a habit or pattern, or take physical activity to an edge that is not sustainable
- increasing awareness of thoughts, feelings and actions
- finding pleasure in new experiences that are available now
- awareness of different reactions, including the protective (fight/flight/

freeze) reaction and the driven Doing mode that can, if overdone, exacerbate the boom-and-bust nature of the condition

- noticing choice points rather than following habitual patterns or expectations from self and others
- setback management planning: noticing precipitating factors, self-care during a setback and ways out of it, using the resources developed as part of self-management and mindfulness
- potential for improved concentration and focus
- collective experience and hearing others' stories and insights and being in a group that understands not just the health condition but also the challenges of self-management and the enforced change in priorities that may ensue.

Linking mindfulness and self-management

The pyramid in Figure 6.1 is a diagrammatic representation of how NICE recommend people with ME/CFS, fibromyalgia and Long Covid are helped. There is a foundation phase where not only medical and diagnostic matters are attended to, but financial, employment and social issues are also addressed. This is being further acknowledged in the UK where from 2022 occupational therapists, physiotherapists and nurses can now write fit notes regarding an individual's ability and needs in returning to work. This is an acknowledgement of the expertise these professions have in ongoing health conditions and in the recovery process.

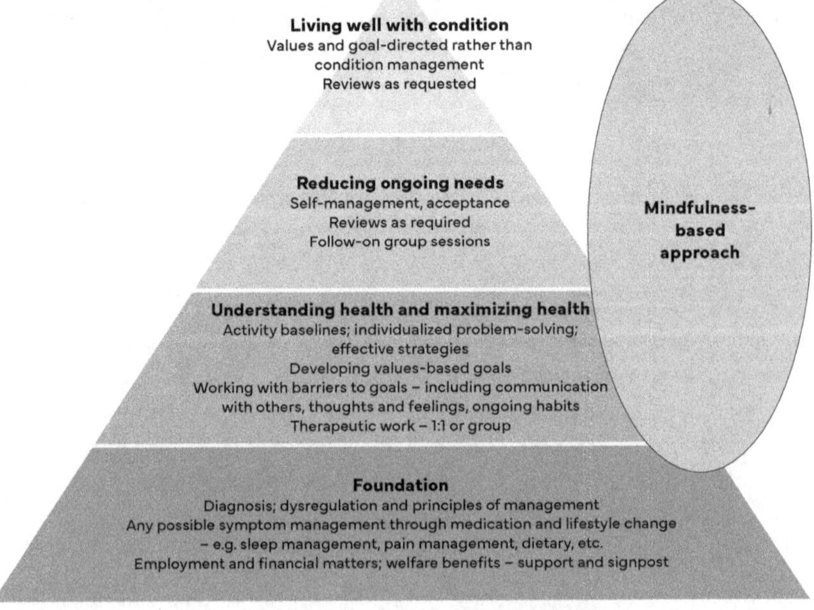

Figure 6.1 Self-management and mindfulness

Mindfulness is represented in an oval that overlaps mainly in the second level of the pyramid, where it can be used as an active therapy and is taught as part of the overall self-management programme. A mindfulness-based approach can support the regulating in the foundation phase; however, its full value is perhaps in providing a way in to an embodied sense of self-management, moment by moment, to addressing the thoughts and feelings that can hamper, and to acknowledging what and who are helpful. As the pyramid rises up to its point, there is less contact with health professionals, but effective self-management includes accessing appropriate help at times as things change or challenges arise.

SUMMARY

So far we have considered self- management and how mindfulness can map onto and support people. It is worth summarizing the situation that people with persistent pain, fatigue and other symptoms are in a complex situation:

- The mindfulness-based approach maps onto and supports symptoms and the self-management of complex situations.
- The complexity is not just in the symptoms and psychological reactions; social and economic factors also require support and need addressing.
- The programme teaches practices to regulate, which can support the stabilizing of physiological patterns.
- Acceptance of the condition and the need to make changes can be observed and acted upon.
- Mindfulness offers a way of inhabiting very small moments of day-to day-life that can be transformative.
- The emphasis on the here and now allows for changes and developments in the individual use of strategies.

Chapter 7

Managing Cognitive Challenges

BRAIN FOG AND MINDFULNESS

- Cognitive processes affected by fatigue
- How mindfulness can support people with their cognitive function
- How the course and associated materials and processes required to do the course can be accessed by people with variable cognitive challenges

Cognitive difficulties reported by people with fatigue

Cognitive difficulties are a main symptom of ME/CFS, post-viral fatigue syndrome and fibromyalgia; the 2021 ME/CFS NICE guideline included it as a key symptom (NICE 2021c). It is often called brain fog and is also reported in post Covid-19 syndrome (NICE 2021a).

'Brain fog' is a shorthand that people use to describe difficulties with concentration, attention, word-finding, short-term memory, mental stamina and speed of mental processing. Some 70–90% of people with ME/CFS and fibromyalgia report cognitive symptoms. It is likely that a similar number with Long Covid will report this too. Other people with conditions, such as those undergoing chemotherapy (chemo brain), menopause, lupus and progressive neurological conditions, report the cognitive symptoms as having a significant impact on their daily lives.

Studies in ME/CFS and fibromyalgia do not suggest these cognitive problems are due to brain damage, and there is little to no evidence that there is an organic problem; long-term memory is not usually affected, nor is cognitive function progressively declining. If there are signs of this, then further neurological testing is required. What we would expect is a variable cognitive picture due to post-exertional symptom exacerbation (Shepherd and Chaudhuri 2020).

A systematic review of ME/CFS and fibromyalgia found that cognitive difficulties were more prevalent than in healthy subjects and that coexisting fatigue, depression, anxiety and pain contributed to, but did not entirely account for, the severity of cognitive symptoms (Teodoro, Edwards and Isaacs 2018).

The systematic review found discrepancies and inconclusive findings in the research studies that my reading felt may be accounted for by post-exertional malaise (therefore variable performance) and the potential for sub-groups of patients with different experiences.

Another systematic review of imaging studies reviewed 63 scientific articles on brain-imaging studies of ME/CFS and concluded that the 'qualitative synthesis of these articles [is] consistent with autonomic dysfunctions in ME/CFS, potentially arising centrally'. In addition, this review highlighted that more extensive brain areas were recruited during cognitive tasks in patients with ME/CFS (Shan et al. 2020). This supports the 'alarm system' theory suggested in chapter 3.

Patients in fatigue clinics routinely report significant problems with cognitive tasks, and part of the educational component at the start of self-management programmes is to help people understand that it is part of the condition and not part of something else. Many people (and their families) are concerned they might be getting dementia as the memory and detail of everyday life is so challenging.

What enables effective cognitive function – a simple description

The brain is a series of complex brain networks working together, and while we categorize the functions of these networks into discrete areas, it can help to label specific functions:

- Thinking speed
- Attention/concentration
- Memory
- Language
- Executive function or fluid intelligence (the ability to reason, learn and apply understanding)
- Crystallized intelligence (knowledge of facts, vocabulary, etc.).

These networks function best when able to flow in a coordinated and aligned way, and the optimal conditions are when calm, as this allows more of the brain to work. However, the system's function is prioritized for survival: if there is a threat, either internal or external, then the systems will prioritize dealing with threat over other mental processes. Therefore, stress, fatigue, pain, fear and any challenges take up space and brain energy, which means the systems are not able to work fluidly. As we currently think that these conditions are due to the body's protective system continuing to 'protect' despite there being no ongoing pathogen or threat, it is understandable that the brain's capacity to manage is chronically affected. This also makes sense of why people can feel they have managed their stress, and may be having treatment for anxiety, but have ongoing problems as their brain remains on 'high alert'.

Pressure to perform will affect us all individually, and all of us function best by going at our own brain's speed. As fatiguing conditions follow a 'boom and bust' pattern, the impact on cognition can be highly variable, and it is common for people to identify that a mentally based activity (answering emails, filling in a form, etc.) can feel as fatiguing as a high-level physical activity. Learning to pace mental activity is part of the skill required, and finding a way to unhook from mental activity and switch to a different mode of activity can help this. For example, spending 15 minutes on a computer-based task, then wiping down the kitchen tops before resting for 20 minutes.

It can be helpful to think of cognitive function as a hierarchy (Figure 7.1); at the base is the survival need to deal with threat stress, illness and pain and this will affect all other processes. The next is the ability to attend or focus. This is a variable component in everyone and highly vulnerable to disruption. It impacts upon all other areas of cognition as we need to be able to attend to something in order to remember it, process it and use it. There are broadly three types of attention:

- Sustained – attending to one thing for a period of time (e.g. reading a book, watching a film)
- Focused/selective (e.g. driving a car)
- Divided (e.g. cooking tea and helping a child with homework).

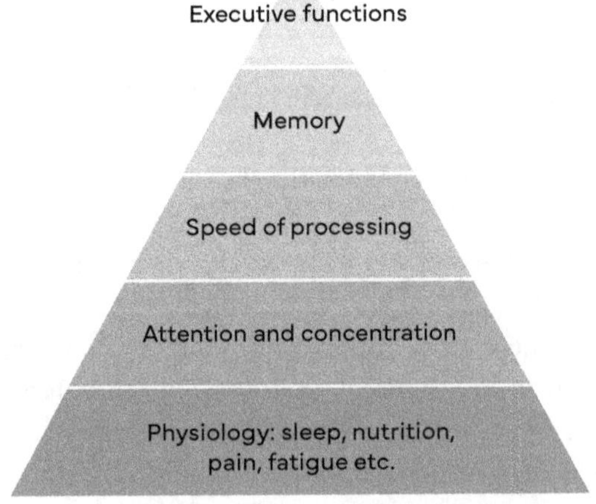

Figure 7.1 Cognitive management hierarchy

The ability to attend impacts on the speed of processing and memory. In order for us to create and retrieve memory there are several stages to the process, simplified as:

- Encoding – getting information into the brain
- Storage – keeping the information there
- Retrieval – accessing the information when needed.

Most people will describe difficulty remembering appointments, conversations or what happened a few days ago, particularly topics that are mundane or repetitive. Memory difficulties are often related to difficulties with attention, which particularly affects the encoding stage – if we cannot attend fully, we are unlikely to encode so well. If there are other factors that impact, such as pain or stress, then that will interrupt attention and therefore other processes.

The strategies to support cognitive fatigue use the hierarchy and start at the bottom and work up with education about the nature of the cognitive problems. For example, knowing that there is no brain damage but that the brain fog is due to a challenge to the brain being able to resource itself and access its networks fully. Perhaps seeing it as a software rather than a hardware problem.

Management

Management of cognitive fatigue is very much embedded in the self-management approach. People sometimes want to 'brain train' using apps; but while these can be enjoyable, on their own they are likely to increase fatigue. A more holistic approach needs to be used, and (once established) concentration techniques could be tried:

- Physiological management: sleep, rest and activity management, nutrition, etc.; stress management; baselines (see chapter 4) and pacing – and the need to pace mental activity as much as physical (e.g. scheduled time to fill in a form)
- Learning how to mentally rest (mindfulness practices can help)
- Being aware of own vulnerabilities and finding ways to address those (e.g. finding it difficult to help child with homework and cook tea, so need to have made tea earlier or delegate the task).

KEY STRATEGIES (DEVELOPED IN A PATIENT-LED PROBLEM SOLVE)

- Acknowledge you are struggling
- Notice if there is too much going on (internally and externally)
- Do one thing at a time
- Prepare your brain and body (breathing, stretching)
- Split tasks into chunks and stop before you can't go on – 'stop before you drop'; 'quit while you are ahead'
- Take the strain off the brain – use notes, reminders on your phone, diaries
- Use your mind for what is important/enjoyable to you (don't 'brain train' unless you really enjoy it)
- Deal with stress
- Say no
- Plan, prioritize, pace
- Ask for help – share tasks, delegate
- Use timers
- Reduce distractions
- Try a reading window on the page.

Mindfulness and cognitive fatigue

A mindfulness-based approach can help with all levels of the cognitive management hierarchy. As discussed in the chapters on the self-management approach (chapters 4 and 6), the contextual factors and how we approach activity is key.

Working with environmental, physiological and stress factors

What are the things that are impacting on ability to attend? Is it stress about finance? Is it too much multi-tasking? Is it poor sleep? Pain? Digestive problems? Sensory overload? Mindful awareness can offer a gentle way to acknowledge and tend to what is here by taking care of oneself and then seeing if there is a way through this, perhaps getting more information, finding another way, not doing something. To 'pause and anchor' can be very helpful here. The conversation or inquiry after each practice is crucial to unhook from the expectation that mindfulness will 'work', and developing the skill of seeing what is going on and being able to resource oneself in the moment, finding ways to respond rather than react and noticing the habitual patterns of activity and mind. Noticing both what stresses and drains us is explored in detail in Session 7 of the course; however, the process of noticing this and building resources is threaded through the course from the first session (see chapter 17 for descriptions of the weekly sessions).

As participants learn to stop, find anchors, ground and explore ways to take care of themselves, they may identify a need to reduce mental activity for a while. Individuals may notice they cannot watch TV, they cannot do all the email and communication they would like, they cannot read a book – if they wish to learn the mindfulness practices as well. Finding time when one is not excessively exhausted may take time. At first, all this can be stressful, so needs to be worked with tenderly by participants and therapists, but can also be liberating as what can be managed becomes apparent.

Attention

Mindfulness practices use sustained, focused and divided attention in the practices. Having an explicit intention to attend in a particular way can be both useful and soothing. Sustaining attention on the breath or on the body in a body scan builds attentional capacity, while people are encouraged to go at their own pace, gently so as not to agitate the system. We offer shorter practices to encourage participation and a sense of achievement that can be built on. It is possible to immediately start work on the capacity to attend, and one exercise we introduce early in the course is a way to work with attention (see box).

FOCUSED ATTENTION PRACTICE
Ten-second exercise to use when you want
to focus or remember something

- Stop (wherever you are).
- Find your feet, take a deep breath.
- Make your body 10% more comfortable.
- Breathe.
- Reflect on what you want to remember/focus on by gently paying attention.
- Is it something someone has said?
- Something you have thought?
- An image?
- A feeling?
- Place your attention on what you wish to focus on for ten seconds.
- If you wish, make a note; do it after you have done this (you will make a better note and it will go in as you are using more of your brain to pay attention).

Divided attention in mindfulness practice

People identify that there can be many things going on in the moment and they can experience them all – irritation at a sound next door while experiencing pleasure in the birds at the bird feeder. One participant described experiencing a headache but could enjoy the feeling of the breath flowing through the body, and by doing this found the pain less intrusive. By practising like this, it becomes possible to intentionally apply this to daily activity as we become used to attending, then intentionally shifting attention to something else. This may have functional carry-over, but also means that it is easier to pace mental activity – I am typing this, I stop and intentionally place my attention on an email and then decide to give my brain a rest and go for a short walk.

Presenting information

The human brain can only hold so much information and has a clever way of organizing connected and complex ideas into packages or bundles that we can usefully recall and share with others. All daily life is organized into this – 'I am going shopping for food' is a shortcut for a range of complex activity, as is 'the chancellor is announcing a budget'. We use chunks to understand what is going on and consider what we may individually do with the information. Each of us will have very different responses according to our previous experience and the circumstances at a particular time (Pinker 2015). How I understand the above statements has varied over time and my response has changed accordingly. For instance, my response to the chancellor announcing the budget today as a health professional and parent in my 50s has changed from when I was studying political history in my 20s.

When people are adapting to changes that have happened due to their ill health, then noticing that they may need to adapt their 'information chunks' is part of accepting and managing their situation. Noticing when they are using 'chunks' that no longer serve them, inquiring into the moment and making understanding explicit can be a useful way to support this. For example, in a group recently there was a discussion about 'physical activity', which for some meant any task that involved some physical effort (e.g. walking upstairs, having a shower, gardening, etc.). For a couple though, 'physical activity' meant exercise: weights at the gym or running. Any other activity was not regarded as 'physical'. The shorthand we use can cause problems as we may use the same words but they have entirely different meanings. As Churchill said when comparing the UK and USA: two nations divided by a common language.

By clarifying and asking and exploring what is meant, the hinterland to a statement like 'physical activity' can be explored. This is looked at in more detail in chapters 12, 14 and 15 on movement and rest.

Additionally, when teaching, considering how information can be easily understood, encoded and accessed is important, particularly with a population who may be struggling to comprehend and retain information. Repeated refrains such as 'responding instead of reacting' and 'how can I take care of myself?' are ways of developing new approaches to their lives. Metaphors such as the two arrows (chapter 5), 'sailing through the window of tolerance' (chapter 9), the 'hot air balloon' (chapter 14) and 'the pit' (chapter 14) enable a shorthand to be created that can be used as a shared experience within the group and beyond. I have had a follow-up session with someone in a flare-up; by being able to access the pit metaphor she remembered what was useful and said at the end, 'We have shone a torch around my pit and I can see how I can start to find the bottom rung.' People talk about improved 'tacking skills' in the window of tolerance (see chapter 9). This active use of metaphor to apply a complex array of self-management techniques is important and refers us back to one of the implicit intentions of mindfulness-based programmes. We are developing a sense of self that is changing and developing rather than remaining with a fixed sense of identity, which, as we have seen, can lead to struggle and suffering.

Developing concentration

Concentration is not actively taught on the course (as it stands); however, some people find their concentration is improved by anchoring and soothing and by the sustained nature of the practices and wish to build on their skills. They then become interested in developing a concentration practice that can then be applied to other activities. It is worth noting that concentration practices are not mindfulness (which is awareness); they are a separate form of meditation that of themselves can be soothing and enable mindful awareness, so it can be a virtuous circle that more mindfulness and peace can be developed by practising concentration. This practice is offered at the end of the course in individual sessions to those who wish to focus on increasing their concentration.

CONCENTRATION PRACTICE

- Settle body and mind (come out of fight/flight). Minimize distractions, phone, etc.
- Choose an object of attention – e.g. a plant, a piece of music, sensation in hands, breath.
- Set a timer – start small (5 minutes).
- Settle your attention gently, become absorbed in your object of attention. When the mind wanders, relax your body and come back to the object. Be gentle.
- Concentration can be relaxing too.

- Practise regularly. Also notice when it's harder – times of day, what's going on?, particular mood, etc. Take care of yourself. Go at your brain's pace.
- Try with other (more complex) activities – e.g. reading, cooking, weeding.

Accessing the course

Some people we work with have times when they cannot read or understand spoken words and enabling the content to be accessed has been a consideration. Meeting the highly variable cognitive needs of people who live with fatigue has been an important consideration. The information is paced, and we have found the use of images and worksheets rather than pages of written ideas important. This led to us splitting the written material into a workbook that gave information about the practice and a separate workbook with information to support the session. The practice log was changed to have less detail, as many reported it was overwhelming and they didn't understand it or do it.

We have tried to ensure that the mindfulness courses go at people's pace, use experiential methods rather than presenting information and emphasize stabilizing and resourcing prior to focusing on attention. Considering environment and location is a factor when managing cognitive fatigue – simple comfortable surroundings and a reduction in interruptions where possible. Going at one's own pace and respecting cognitive capacity in the session and during home practice is crucial. We try to encourage people to come even if it is a bad day; this is easier on Zoom as they sometimes log in for the practice at the beginning with the camera off and then either just listen to the group session or log off. We ask that they let us know what they are doing.

For many this is a new way of doing things and there can be carry-over into other areas. For example, Kairi: 'I am now able to let my daughter have a friend around even if I don't feel well. Previously, I avoided anyone being here or interacting when I was on a bad day as I struggle to speak or think.'

SUMMARY

- Brain fog affects the ability to focus, attend, find words, plan and carry out tasks. In fatiguing conditions, it can be highly variable and distressing and confusing for both the person with the health condition and those around them.
- Self-management is hierarchical, first focusing on contextual and environmental factors and considering stress, pain, medication and sleep.

- 'Brain training' such as attention or memory games will not help improve things without the contextual factors, and in many cases it is better to take the strain off the brain with lists, prompts and delegation. However, if brain training is relaxing and enjoyable, it could well be helpful.
- Mindfulness can help manage stress reaction; awareness enables the contextual factors to be observed and choices made – 'how can I take care of myself?'
- Meditation can be used to develop concentration; while this is not mindfulness, it can support mindful awareness.
- The cognitive problems with fatigue mean that the practices and the educational information are designed for a range of cognitive abilities.
- The sessions are flexible and people are very much encouraged to attend 'as they are'.

Chapter 8

Underlying Processes in Mindfulness Programmes

- Modes of mind – Being and Doing modes that underpin how we think and feel
- Three emotional regulation systems
- How fatiguing health conditions can impact how we emotionally regulate, and how we soothe may need to change because of health conditions
- Mindful awareness of which mode or system we are in and using this awareness to make choices
- How the emotional regulation systems are taught throughout the programme

While it is tempting to see ourselves as unique individuals and indeed we all have a unique expression of genes, experience and context, there are different modes we end up operating within that drive our thoughts, feelings and behaviours. These are not errors or things to be corrected, rather they are part of how we have evolved as a species, particularly how our brain and nervous system has evolved. Understanding these processes is an explicit part of mindfulness programmes.

Modes of mind

Recognizing that we have different modes of mind is a key principle in mindfulness-based cognitive therapy (Crane 2017b; Feldman and Kuyken 2019; Segal et al. 2013). 'Doing mode of mind' refers to the active, problem-solving and goal-directed mode of mind that we use every day to manage day-to-day life and to plan our future. We use our experience and memories to shape what we will do next, either to avoid repeating mistakes or to ensure we repeat success. The Doing mode of mind is very successful at this and is essential to manage a host of things in life. It becomes a problem when we use it to solve problems or work towards desired states that cannot be solved by goal-setting and planning.

Problems such as sadness, despair and the desire for joy and fulfilment cannot be scheduled and organized to happen. Like sleep and rest, we can create conditions for certain states to be more or less likely, but we cannot feel joy nor can we sleep on command.

The other challenge that is a product of our evolution is sometimes termed 'discrepancy-based processing', in which we are constantly evaluating our experience and looking at what we either need to do to get where we want to be or what we ought to be doing. This is an amazing part of humanity; it has led to all sorts of inventions and problems being solved. However, it gives little space to appreciating what we have done, as experiences that are regarded as safe and non-threatening are brushed off and not engaged with by a brain that prioritizes what is necessary for survival. This tendency fuels Doing mode's attempt to solve those problems it cannot solve. This can result in Doing mode of mind working very hard, and what happens is that 'driven doing' mind (stressed and ruminating about what it should be doing) takes over. However, there is another mode of mind that is available to us – Being mode.

Being mode is an experience of this moment where one is absorbed and inhabiting the moment through senses and direct perception. It is not actively trying to feel anything, it is waking up to what is here right now – from awareness of the room temperature to feet on the floor, the sounds of cars in the distance and the rain on the roof. The feeling of tension in my shoulders and then a sense of relief when my cat comes home after two nights out. I may not actively solve problems, but I am aware of how connected I feel to my cat and how that soothes me.

Being mode is actively cultivated with mindfulness through awareness of the smells, texture and taste of the orange I am eating, instead of being lost in thought planning the meal I am going to cook for my mother this evening.

Being mode is available to us all but is rarely the mode we engage without practice. If we have reason to avoid our situation, because it is so difficult, then learning to inhabit it can be tender work. Going back to Sasha in chapter 5, Doing mind predominated her experience, and while wanting to be better, she was aware of the feelings of shame that got in the way of her asking for help. When she told the GP and then the therapist, who responded with understanding and asked more questions that uncovered the full situation, she was surprised that no one thought she was stupid; instead practical measures were initiated. She needed help, and she was emailed phone numbers and had support in how she went about sorting this out but could go at her own pace. This in turn allowed her to contact two friends who astounded her with their support and understanding, although she was aware of profound loss as her family did not understand or feel they could help her. Doing the mindfulness course she was able to notice all of this, but was at times very aware of a huge sense of loss for her job, family and fear for her future. She had regular sessions with the therapist during the course to support her in acknowledging this and focusing on what was resourcing her now, so she wasn't washed away with overwhelm for the past or the future.

Being able to access Being mode of mind enables different parts of the brain to come online, which actually can give us more options (think of Paul in chapter 5 and the options that opened up to him). This, as discussed in the next section, is built on further by understanding that our feelings and behaviour are directed by our biology and that this is a result of our evolution. Understanding this can overlay our understanding and awareness and give us a focus for considered action that has a particular quality.

Emotional regulation systems

Paul Gilbert's work on compassion-focused therapy (Gilbert 2010, 2020; Gilbert and Choden 2013) is based on the way human evolution shapes our feelings and actions. This work has created a deceptively simple framework, and just about everyone we have shown it to immediately understands and can apply it, I think because it describes the texture and tone of the experience. It is considered further in chapter 14 about activity management. This model clusters our emotional responses broadly into three systems explaining some of the biology and considers the ways in which ways of thinking and behaving can both lead to and arise from the system we may be in at the time. Rather than seeing the more tangled and difficult stressful states we are in as something to be 'mended', it sees them as essential to our survival and that our feelings and behaviours are entirely understandable through the lens of human evolution. However, these reactions may not always be helpful given that our world and brains have changed and require adaptive responses. How we can understand and work with our fundamental drives and these systems and cultivate a compassionate response is the basis of compassion-focused therapy. The three-systems model is used (Figure 8.1) within this mindfulness-based approach to support awareness. Understanding which of the systems we are being regulated by can help us understand why we are doing what we are doing. This enables us to notice the reaction, classify it and consider *how* we want to act. This model also allows the cultivation of more desirable states so that we can intentionally improve more helpful parts of our body/mind. Figure 8.1 summarizes the model with the double arrows between each system showing that we move between the systems.

This model includes driven or motivated states as well as the commonly known dual model of fight/flight/freeze vs. relax/digest. The separation of 'doing' into 'threat/protection' and 'drive' helps people identify what feels good and usefully challenges the idea that being calm and rested is always desirable.

Sometimes, we need and want to get things done and going out and about can be vitalizing and pleasurable. Additionally, while rest and digest is part of soothe, this is a wider system encompassing the need for (and the possibility of) connecting to others and feeling safe and calm.

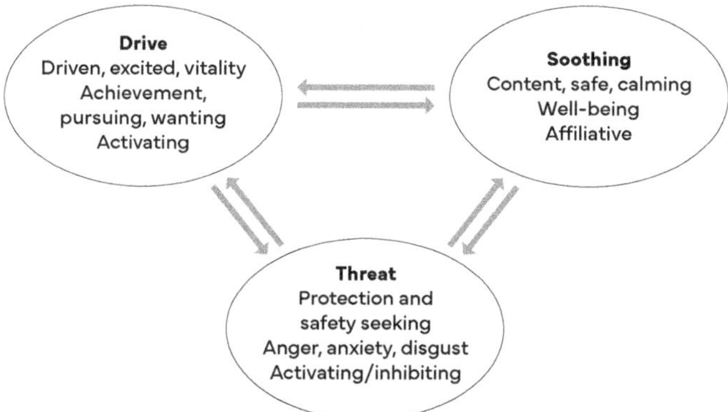

Figure 8.1 Three-systems model of emotional regulation (adapted from Gilbert 2010)

Threat system

This system reacts very quickly in order to protect us from threats and get us to safety. It operates on a 'better safe than sorry' principle, which means it will override pleasure or contentment (Gilbert 2010) and can come online rapidly and at times excessively. This system is part of the sympathetic nervous system and the hypothalamic–pituitary–adrenal (HPA) axis, which both lead to an active response. As discussed in chapter 3, this reaction is the basis of the 'alarm' system that is highly sensitive in people who have fatigue and pain conditions. The Threat system can lead to an activated response (fight or flight), where we run or lash out, or a deactivated response (freeze; for an example of this, think of a mouse playing dead when being played with by a cat).

The emotions associated with threat and protection are anger, anxiety, disgust, fear. The behaviours can lead to conflict but also to overwhelm and a withdrawal. This withdrawal and retreat into activities such as excessive TV watching, alcohol use and ignoring social contact are a protective response. The Threat system can also be activated when there is social isolation, as being connected is a fundamental part of being human and isolation is a threat to survival.

When people are not able to access social networks or activity they enjoy or find satisfying, this will activate Threat. The reduction in ability to socialize or engage in meaningful activity experienced by people who have fatiguing conditions means it is likely many will be in the Threat system for prolonged periods. Additionally, the status of the conditions, the uncertainty of diagnosis and lack of understanding or medical tests can lead people to feel isolated and therefore threatened.

Soothing system

The Soothing system comes 'online' when animals have enough food and are in a safe place. It is also what parents do to offspring when they are distressed; we pick up, cuddle, stroke, nuzzle, and try to make them feel safe. Over time the young learn to do that for themselves and in turn do this for their own offspring. The feelings we have in the Soothing system, such as contentment, connection, affection, and so on, are not achieved by doing things or acquiring something but by feeling supported, appreciated, understood and validated and by experiencing kindness. As we develop, we can learn to do this for ourselves with acts of self-care, kindness and self-compassion. This suggests that 'the soothing system can regulate the threat system and help to calm the emotions we experience when we are in danger such as anxiety, anger and disgust' (Lee and James 2012, p.26).

Drive system

The Drive system enables us to flourish and create. It can help us get the things we need to survive – food, sex, shelter, and a sense of achievement that makes us feel good. Drive means we get things done, make things, problem-solve and have fun. However, too much drive can lead us in to 'driven doing', a sense that there is always more to do, always a way to problem-solve and progress, which can in turn lead us into the Threat system. On the other hand, not enough drive and achievement can leave us feeling lethargic, bored and depressed and again back into Threat.

Movement between the systems

In a regulated system there is a flow; for example, I might be in Soothing having a cup of tea in the garden taking in plants, birdsong and the sky, then I might go into Drive when I go to empty the dishwasher while waiting for my laptop to load my Zoom account for a meeting; then I discover that my bank card has gone missing, which sends me into Threat mode; I then take some deep breaths to soothe myself, then go into Drive while I call the bank, feel better and down-regulate with my cat into Soothing again.

Problems arise when the systems become out of balance, which can happen with chronic illness, pain or prolonged stress. While the drive or achievement system can be fun and we have a sense of achievement, it can also be used to try and manage difficulties that cannot be solved in this way, trying all sorts of things to overcome and problem-solve or distract ourselves away from what is going on. Our culture is very much geared up to this: if we could just find the right exercise, therapist, diet, vitamin supplement, medication, we would be better (and there are many who want to take our money in this process). While all those things can be useful, they are unlikely to solve the basic problem all humans have: life is a struggle and there are challenges we cannot push our way through.

Conditions such as ME/CFS, fibromyalgia and Long Covid don't have an easy answer. Dietary changes, appropriate exercise, meditation and so on can be useful, but so far there is uncertainty about the mechanism for the symptoms and no obvious thing we can do or take. Whatever we 'do' to try and 'fix' it, the problems cannot be solved, and as the struggling increases, so does the suffering. The boom-and-bust cycle can be activated by striving and operating at a level that is no longer sustainable. Failure to solve problems through the Drive mode or by doing more than the individual can manage can lead the body to feel it is threatened and therefore activate the protective system so the muscles and circulatory system become active and ready to fend off what feels like a threat. In people who have a system that is very responsive to these messages, this leads to an increase in symptoms, which affects someone's ability to manage day-to-day tasks and can interrupt plans and routines as the individual then needs to have time to recover. This at best can lead to piling up of tasks to be done, which can escalate to loss of social contact, reduction in income as well as perpetuating weakness and disability.

From the perspective of fatigue management, knowing what we enjoy and find satisfying is important. Many activities, while costing us energy, also give us energy. Sometimes rest is not the answer, and we need to do something different. Appreciating that we are in the Threat mode can help us understand why we pull away and hide. We can identify if there is a more soothing approach that we can start to incorporate into our repertoire of responses. We can start to understand and forgive ourselves, realizing that what we do is the result of not only our personal history, but also how we have evolved as a species. It is how we are built; our reactions are human. Ultimately it is not our fault, but perhaps there is a way we can take care of ourselves, and spotting what is going on is a good start.

Changes due to fatiguing health conditions

People living with debilitating levels of fatigue symptoms that are exacerbated by exertion are often having to learn to inhabit a very new way of living, having to consider what they can do and perhaps do it differently. Their experience of the systems may be very different now to how it was. For example, someone whose idea of relaxing is walking by themselves on long-distance trails, but is now only able to walk 20 metres and uses a wheelchair for longer outings, can find it very hard to engage in activity that soothes or cultivates appropriate levels of drive. Please see chapter 15 on rest for more detail on the changes in perspective that people may be making. Figure 8.2 shows how drive and threat interact to create a stressed or overdriven state in people.

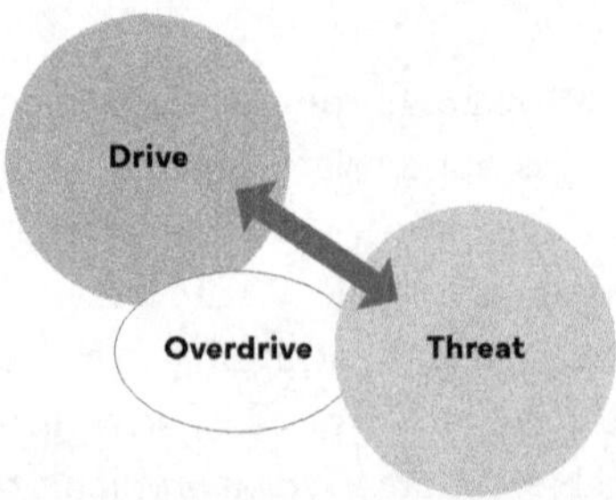

Figure 8.2 How Drive and Threat interact to create a stressed or overdriven state

If threat is activated and it is hard to access Soothing or appropriate levels of Drive, the boom-and-bust patterns of activity seen in chronic health conditions can be exacerbated, as shown in Figure 8.3.

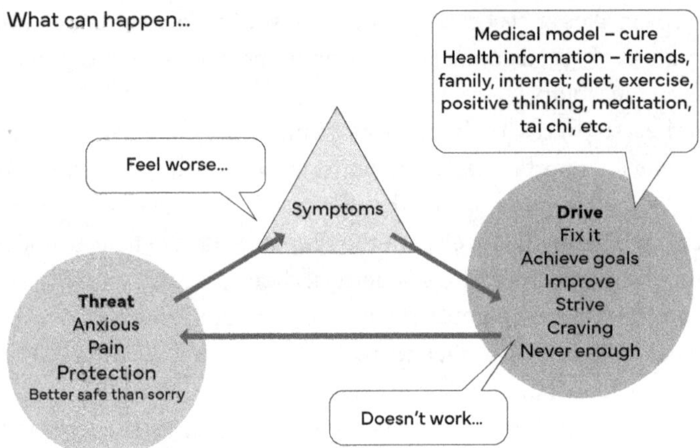

Figure 8.3 How the rest and drive systems can exacerbate
the challenge in managing a health condition

The Soothing system as well as regulating Threat can be how we could appreciate all we do in the Drive system. We can notice and acknowledge the window box we have weeded, the meal we have prepared, the report we have written, and acknowledge either the pleasure of having the meal and the attractive window box or the sense of achievement that we have finished the report (or at least the pleasure at being able to do something else now). Being able to appreciate what one has done becomes very important if activity is being managed and done differently.

Going back to Paul in chapter 5, knowing that he had overexerted with housework but that he could plan a different evening with his boyfriend required planning and problem-solving. It also enhanced the Soothing system and made the conditions possible for greater connection as he was able to connect with Tim as he was and potentially be validated and understood, which would increase their connection and soothing.

This can be tender and delicate work as people navigate not only how they feel about the changes they need to make, but also how those around them feel and how they are accepted and validated.

Figure 8.4 shows how the Soothing system can regulate both Drive and Threat.

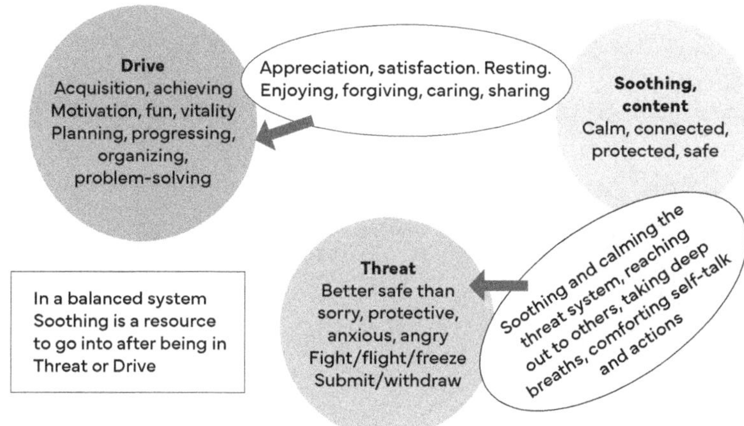

Figure 8.4 How Soothing can moderate Threat and Drive

For people with health conditions who are ascertaining how much is enough, the use of activity goals and baselines can support Drive being accessed in a useful way (see chapters 4, 6 and 14 for more detail). This can develop a sense of self-efficacy and confidence that optimizes this system. Additionally, by having realistic and meaningful goals that match current capacity, drive is developed and it gives time and capacity for reflection. This reflection can include appreciation and acknowledgement, which is part of the Soothing system. We can connect to ourselves and offer soothing to ourselves, which in turn means we are more likely to be able to offer this to others, which sets up the potential for reciprocity with others. Kindness begets kindness. Drive being accessed in a useful way is shown in Figure 8.5.

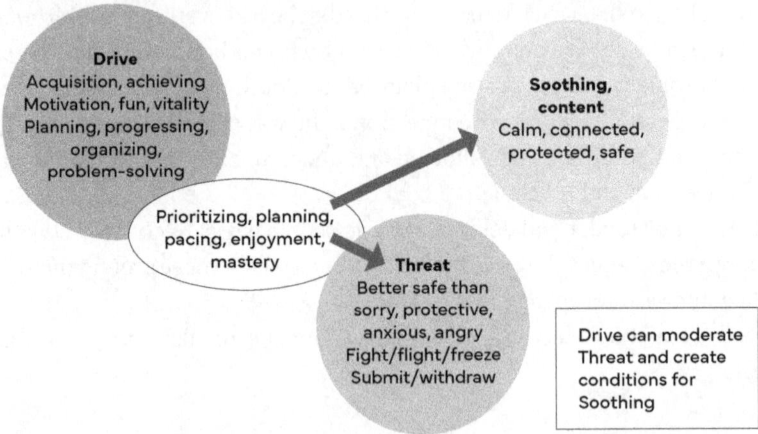

Figure 8.5 Drive can moderate Threat and create conditions for Soothing

All three systems are connected and Figure 8.6 shows the links between them.

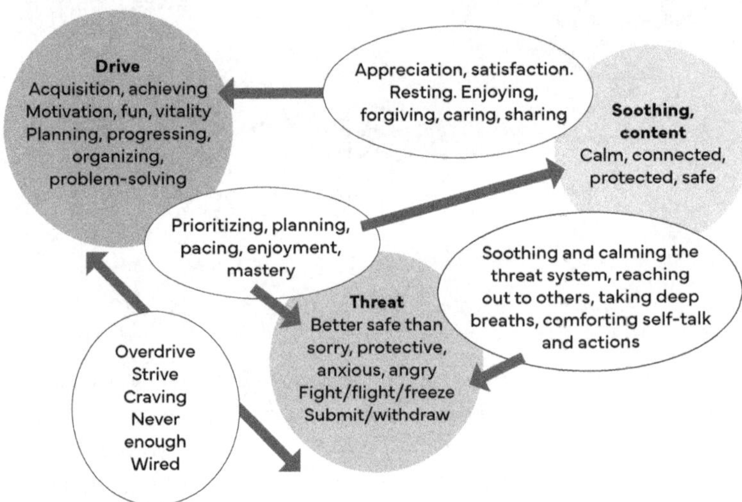

Figure 8.6 How the systems interact

Mindfulness practice

The practice component of the programme enables emotional regulation concepts to be taught experientially as awareness is developed. But as well as promoting awareness of the systems and what may be regulating or deregulating us, the practices provide a way to access the Soothing system and Being mode of mind. Mindfulness practices are exactly what they say – practice at purposely paying attention in a particular way. The course builds from being aware of the moment and finding ways to settle and ground and then gently increasing awareness and being with the present moment as it is. As the course progresses there is an invitation to turn towards more difficult matters with the skill of grounding and being able to soothe. However, this is not mere rehearsal for the show; by practising, one is cultivating a particular mode of mind that is of itself calming, soothing and less reactive, so enabling one to pay better attention. These are functions of the executive centre of the brain that regulates and recognizes emotions and is where we plan and organize and 'think'. This organizing part of the brain enables us to be aware of options and to make considered choices. It is also where we experience empathy by being able to imagine how another person might feel or act and how we may feel and act in the future. It is where we reflect (Gilbert 2020; Gilbert and Choden 2013; Lee and James 2012).

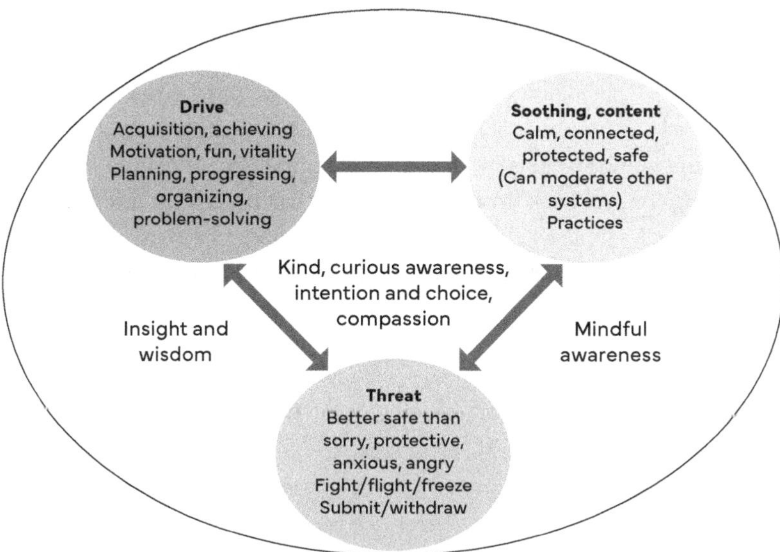

Figure 8.7 Mindful awareness and attitudes of the three emotional regulation systems

The capacity to 'witness' ourselves and take care of ourself in the moment requires the ability to stop, observe and respond. Understanding that we have fundamental systems that can be running and directing our thoughts, feelings and actions, and that those systems are a key part of our biology and human development, means we can access this more observational place and choose how we respond. It also means we can understand when we are reactive and understand where that comes from, increasing the opportunity for self-care and soothing. Having the support and understanding of others, and also giving support to others, enhances the connection and therefore the Soothing system. However, this is not necessarily straightforward as we can also become aware of the more difficult memories, and going gently is important. Being able to notice when things are difficult and overwhelming and going at one's own pace is key. A common pitfall is to identify mindfulness with soothing, and while it can enhance soothing, it is primarily an awareness of all the systems. Figure 8.7 attempts to show that mindful awareness of the systems and the flow between the systems, with particular emphasis on attitudes such as curiosity, friendly awareness and the possibility of wise choices.

How the systems are taught through the mindfulness programme

The systems are formally introduced in Week 4, but they are alluded to in the earlier sessions and practices. Preparing participants so they feel connected and grounded and have some control is intended to help them access the regulating, executive part of their brain, so learning mindfulness practices is as fruitful as they can be. This includes the initial orientation to the group in individual appointments and group sessions (see chapter 16). The group processes support soothing and going at one's own pace, so we purposely do not go around the room asking for feedback. In the inquiry into the practice, there is always a recognition that people will have different experiences and a curiosity as to how people took care of themselves, soothed themselves in the moment. When we are in a physical room there are choices in chair, cushions, etc., and there is an invitation to experiment and move as much as required. While we encourage people to manage themselves, support can be offered. Participants often help each other too, although this is navigated as we have a group agreement not to offer advice and help unless this is requested.

The practices at the beginning focus on being able to pause, stop and feel into physical support *before* we bring awareness; this is to bring the Soothing system online so the awareness has a curious and gentle quality. This is an embodied approach, using the body as a resource through movement, positioning and adjustment.

The Soothing system is overtly introduced in Sessions 2 and 3. In Session 2, we spend time thinking what will help, both in the group and between sessions using the window of tolerance (Siegel 1999) and an immediate application of principles into daily activity.

This knowledge is developed in Session 3 with the awareness of a pleasant events activity by initially bringing awareness to the Soothing system and the activities that can support and develop soothing. There is an invitation to make pleasant things happen either through noticing what is pleasant or by actively doing something one finds pleasant (Germer 2009).

Awareness of being able to actively control and direct as well as respond to what happens sets up some resources for being able to actively move towards more challenging experience, but with an awareness of both a choice that 'I can do this' and that there are resources available to manage 'even if it is really hard'. The homework practice of recording reactions to small unpleasant (annoying) events gives people a sense of appreciation of what they already do to manage and how the small things can add up to a sense of increased regulation. There is often surprise and relief at the practice of turning towards difficulty, as the pressure of not looking or making things OK all the time and monitoring for when it is not OK is exhausting and stressful.

The Threat system is introduced in Session 4 through the inquiry into unpleasant events, and at this point we name all three systems and consider how the Drive and Threat systems can work together in the boom-and-bust activity cycle.

In Session 5, the Threat system is explored further by noticing the body's reaction in the 'Sea of reaction' exercise (Bartley 2011). There is an automatic tendency to withdraw, tense and spiral as our thinking and behaviour is regulated by the protective response. Considering how one behaves in that reaction and how typical that might be is useful. It can suggest the possibility that there might be other ways and that the Drive system can be usefully employed to plan and organize alternatives.

Being gently aware and finding choice points is a theme developed in Session 6 in looking at the role of thoughts, and Session 7 brings awareness to Drive-based activities, things that bring us mastery and enjoyment and continue to express the motif we have used throughout the course: *What do I need to do now? And how do I need to do it based on what I know?*

This awareness of the Threat system, the potential challenge of the Soothing system and the capacity to become aware of what is or has been difficult is potentially destabilizing. The next chapter considers how a trauma-informed approach is folded into the programme.

SUMMARY

- Mindful awareness is cultivated through paying attention to the present moment; however, this moment is complex, and having an awareness of processes and states of mind emotion is challenging.
- The modes of mind in MBCT offer a way to identify how we are approaching our experience; are we in 'Doing mode'? This is where we fix, organize and problem-solve, which can be helpful, but when it is applied to challenges such as low mood and fatigue or problems that cannot be easily remedied, it can increase stress and a sense of difficulty.

- 'Being mode of mind' allows a more expansive and curious and less judgemental state to arise that can allow us to soothe and also enables the mind to make more creative choices and tend to the challenge of the situation rather than try to make it stop.
- The three emotional regulation systems (Gilbert 2009) are a way of mapping different emotional regulation systems and how we move between them.
- Mindful awareness offers a way to observe how we are and to cultivate alternative, perhaps more compassionate and creative, states.

Chapter 9

Resourcing and Regulating

TRAUMA-INFORMED PRACTICE

- Trauma-informed practice in mindfulness-based approaches
- Links between trauma and fatigue
- Trauma-informed strategies to support people learning mindfulness for fatigue

Trauma-informed practice in mindfulness-based approaches

One of the challenges of mindful awareness is that this awareness can lead to a feeling of overwhelm. Understanding that driven doing and the Threat system can be running the show is one thing, but having the skills to self-care or self-regulate is another. Many people will have had experiences that have left their nervous systems hyper-vigilant (Porges 2007; van der Kolk 2014). Settling, stillness and awareness can lead to a feeling of unease at best or escalate into being triggered and having to deal with unwanted memories and a fight/flight/freeze reaction: 'when we invite someone with trauma to pay attention to their internal world, we invite them into contact with traumatic stimuli – thoughts, images, memories and physical sensations that may relate to a traumatic event' (Treleaven 2018, p.6).

In response to some of the difficulties, David Treleaven and others have explored and developed trauma-sensitive mindfulness training for mindfulness teachers as well as clinicians. The book *Essential Resources for Mindfulness Teachers* (Crane et al. 2021) summarizes this work and outlines how trauma sensitivity can be useful for everyone, and good practice is to fold trauma sensitivity into all programmes. This includes how the group is paced and organized, how the teacher relates to the group and the practice, and how the practices and other exercises are guided (Gold in Crane et al. 2021, pp.184–186).

Trauma and fatigue

As discussed in chapter 3, we understand the symptoms of fatigue to be part of a dysregulated protective reaction whereby the fight/flight/freeze response is readily activated with normally benign input. This can be either because the person has a strong predisposition through genetic or early childhood experiences (de Venter et al. 2017; Espeleta et al. 2020; Helm et al. 2009) and/or because they have been ill with a virus or other infection or injury and/or a stressful period of time that means the protective reaction is on most or all of the time, which means the body does not rest. Additionally, the process by which people become ill and are impacted by the consequences of the condition can be highly activating. If you weren't stressed before, you are understandably feeling it now. Mindfulness programmes need to bear this in mind and consider:

- how people are taken into the group
- the environment in which the course is taught; the relationship between the facilitator and the group
- the relationships between group members
- the way the practices are taught.

The mindfulness practices have been adapted to take into account and actively work with the challenges created by fatigue, particularly cognitive challenges and pain, and so on. The additional problems due to the fluctuating, or boom-and-bust, pattern of symptoms and activity can be further activating. Trauma-informed mindfulness offers a way in which the overactive Threat system can intrude on how people rest and manage their daily activities.

The mindfulness practices in our course initially focus on learning to regulate and directly teach people about the role of regulation as development of education about the 'alarm system' and dysregulation model (see chapter 3). Session 2 has been restructured and named 'Resourcing ourselves'. This is initially done experientially during the inquiry into the body scan in the session and in the homework review. Attention is drawn to how people are currently managing and how they are already regulating throughout their day. For example, they may find the body scan uncomfortable but notice that they opened their eyes and moved, and that made it feel better. In the week, they may have found there were times when the practice was not comfortable and chose a different time or place where it felt more easeful.

Participants are also learning to stop and perhaps actively relax and rest, but this can be problematic as it can feel as though they are 'getting it wrong' if they don't feel a particular way. This is a fine line to balance, and the neutral yet interested stance of the group leader in inquiring into all experience and being interested in whatever it is counters a goal-focused approach to learning to relax or regulate. By learning to notice when we react and how we helpfully respond meets the course intention as a pragmatic intervention in self-management.

As therapists/mindfulness teachers, we also need to know when we are activated and to have a sense of when we are reacting, and we need to understand how we regulate ourselves. Continuing to practise and seeking help for the tender points in our own lives is part of the work. Noticing how we react or respond to difficulties may not be shared overtly, but will increase our capacity to compassionately inquire, listen and be present for those we are intending to help. Please see *Essential Resources for Mindfulness Teachers* (Crane et al. 2021) for more detail on this.

The window of tolerance

The 'window of tolerance' refers to a zone of optimal physiological functioning where the individual is not so over-aroused as to feel agitated, anxious and hyper-vigilant, and is not so under-aroused that they are lethargic, withdrawn and depressed (Siegel 1999).

The image of sailing through the window of tolerance (Figure 9.1) provides a useful metaphor, while echoing the boom-and-bust pattern of symptoms seen in fatiguing health conditions (Unity Health n.d.).

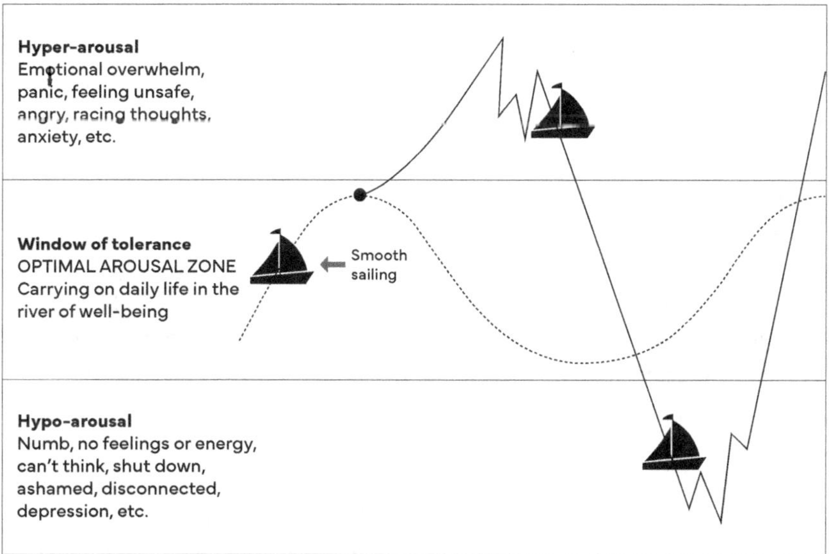

Figure 9.1 Sailing through the window of tolerance (with permission from Unity Health)

The window can vary depending on psychological and physiological factors and can be 'widened' with awareness and regulation skills. The metaphor of sailing is useful as it introduces an active process that can be related to and used immediately: we all navigate and have times when things can feel easier than at other times when we can feel anxious or overwhelmed. The image is of sailing through different waters, noticing the calm waters but also having some skills to navigate the choppy seas, in much the way a sailor learns their craft. This metaphor is useful as it implies that there will be rough seas and they can be difficult and feel dangerous, but perhaps there are ways of managing them rather than having to avoid the choppy waters altogether, which reduces our capacity to be involved and travel to different places.

How the window of tolerance can help

It is important that we do not feel that we must cope all the time (as some storms are too great or perhaps our ship needs some maintenance, is worn out, etc.) and can ask for help (perhaps we need a fleet?), and this is overtly discussed. We use this metaphor on the course to initially help people notice what they are already doing to sail through, what resources are already present, and how we can pay attention to those as much as the difficult feelings. Knowing our resources can help us through the difficult times, and the mindfulness group can be a way to try them out on things that don't matter, the practices are really that – practices.

Sailing through the window of tolerance is introduced early to support any problems that may arise with developing increased awareness. A problem that can arise early in the programme is that people don't feel relaxed and immediately feel they are doing it wrong. As well as helping someone explore the reaction and what is challenging, the idea of 'tacking' through rougher seas is explored, and as much or more time is spent noticing what helps and also intentionally adding in activity that does help, such as opening eyes, shifting attention, moving, getting a drink. One does not have to 'stay with' strong challenging feelings that increase aversion and stress and hang out there; it is important that we tend to the feelings and take care of ourselves, gently building resources and skills. Please see chapter 11 on inquiry for an example of this. By tending to feelings of aversion, through noticing and making shifts with an attitude of care and consideration, the idea is that the window of tolerance can increase. Mindfulness, by actively tending to difficulty, without going into Threat mode, then noticing how the moment can change, can support the expansion of the window of tolerance without pressure. If one is feeling pressure to be any other way than how one is, this can be noticed and tended to as well.

Group leaders can support people managing challenge by being available for the participants; for example, by welcoming contact with any questions and highlighting in the intake individual sessions that getting in touch with a problem is part of the programme. Occasionally, there is a need to contact someone directly after the session. Sometimes this means that it is agreed the programme is at the wrong time for the individual and they may need alternative support or the practices can be adapted. Giving choice about length of practices and which practices, and developing a sense of curiosity about what they are noticing, supports this. For example, we have several people who start with the looking and listening practices instead of the body scans, who use movement of the hands instead of the breath or sensation. People we know who have done this report being able to gradually bring their awareness to their body and find that this can lead to a significant change in how they relate to their symptoms.

The ways in which a trauma-informed approach is managed are considered in chapter 16 on practical considerations.

Turning towards challenge

The idea of tacking through choppy waters and storms seeds the mindfulness concepts of turning towards and accessing compassion for oneself in challenging times. Can we look for what supports and resources us, rather than feel we must cope all the time or have failed if we don't? While looked at in detail in Session 5, the principle is here from the beginning. This image is sometimes referred to later in the course by participants:

> 'I feel I have better tacking skills now, I find my feet, straighten my body when I need to deal with something, but I can also let myself drop and roll out tension from my shoulders rather than brace myself to keep going.'

> 'I'm aware of when I'm in choppy waters or when a storm is brewing and can take steps to move through this.'

The ability or expectation that one can regulate or soothe through challenges needs to be used with some caution as we are trying to be present with what is, not create an alternative state of consciousness (Varela, Thompson and Rosch 2017). Not adding to the experience at all and getting through rather than 'coping' can be the wisest, most compassionate response: 'I'm in stormy waters, it's difficult. I don't like it. How can I take care of myself?'

This visual representation of the window of tolerance is helpful and conceptualizes the intentions of the whole course:

- Highlighting that there can be problems and that awareness can be challenging, but that there are ways to work with this, the course is about developing resources to help in learning to manage this.
- It shows that we can be aware of what helps and supports us as much as we can be aware of what deregulates us, linking existing skills and strategies to the mindfulness programme.

- To learn and support self-regulation and develop the ability to stop and pause and unwind tension or conversely 'up-regulate' if zoning out or going into hypo-arousal.
- Discussing regulation rather than rest or relaxation is important. There can be a desire to feel better through relaxation; changing that to regulation and soothing and considered action is more active and in line with what mindfulness can offer.
- Offering hope that the window of tolerance can be increased and, where it can't, that the challenges can be tended.
- Identifying that the ability to regulate will be variable depending on factors that may be outside of our control, but that it is possible to respond and not be blown around by outside forces or to take care of oneself when this is happening.

This chapter is an example of how we can move from suffering to wise action very quickly with simple measures. The experiential nature of the course means participants can experience this early in the process.

SUMMARY

- The mindfulness programme is intended as a pragmatic intervention to resource the self-management of fatigue syndromes.
- Being able to regulate is a skill that can be developed which can support self-management.
- Many people with fatigue have an activated stress reaction due to the nature of their illness and its sequalae. Some have adverse early life experiences that may have ongoing impact.
- Awareness, stillness and introspection can trigger or exacerbate distress, so practices and processes need to be aware of this and use trauma-informed principles.
- The window of tolerance is a useful visual aid to support people identifying when they are feeling overwhelmed and overstimulated and for developing resources to regulate themselves.

SUMMARY OF PART 1

Part 1 has looked at some of the theoretical underpinnings to mindfulness programmes and how they can apply to people living with fatiguing conditions.

- We are continually reacting to our experience.
- This reaction can disrupt plans, activity, relationships.
- Humans have evolved in particular ways that make these reactions understandable. Illness and trauma can affect this further as the protective system can become dysregulated.
- It is possible to learn ways to respond, but fatiguing health conditions mean that this is complicated as what we can do varies so much.
- Contemplative and cognitive science offer ways of understanding that underpin the mindfulness-based programmes.
- Therapists and mindfulness teachers need to be aware of trauma reactions and consider this in all elements of their practice, from how the group is established through to the individual practices.

PART 2

Mindfulness Practices and Teaching Considerations

ADAPTATION AND NUANCE

The term 'mindfulness practice' is used rather than meditation as we are inviting people to practise a specific task. Meditation is a blanket term for a huge array of activity from visualization to religious practices. As this is a health-based intervention with the specific and explicit intention of supporting people to manage their health condition within the context of the fatigue and pain services, being able to use the practices to manage their particular needs in everyday activity is a key component to the course. This is different to learning to meditate at a Buddhist centre where the act of meditation may have very different intentions and specific goals. In a short programme, it is essential to be clear about what can be learnt, and ascertaining each individual's match for the programme before they start is important.

This mindfulness-based programme for fatigue uses both formal and informal practices. In many ways, the informal may be more important to the people doing this course, as it is how we approach everyday life that makes a difference, and for people living with fatiguing and painful health conditions that may mean finding completely new ways of doing things and also dealing with the loss, guilt, shame and confusion that can arise.

The 'formal' practices provide an opportunity to learn how to be mindful, to practise the approach with an understanding of how the mind works, and to develop resources as insight and compassion grow. By giving time to it and experiencing other ways of responding to habitual patterns, we are more able to do so in daily life. We don't have much evidence about whether the approach helps with or without the formal practice, or about how long one needs to do it for (Strohmaier, Jones and Cane 2021); however, in the prevention of relapse in depression: '...participants who reported that they engaged in formal home practice on at least 3 days a week during the treatment phase were almost half as likely to relapse as those who reported fewer days of formal practice' (Crane et al. 2014).

Feedback from our follow-up groups is that people find it useful to check back in with the formal practice and the approach even if they don't do much formal practice in between.

The practices taught in contemporary mindfulness-based interventions are based on the early Buddhist practices of calm abiding (*samatha*) and insight (*vipassana*) (Wellings 2016). Later Buddhist practices are sometimes included in mindfulness-based programmes, such as the compassion-based practices in, for example, the Breathworks approach to pain and illness (Burch and Penman 2013), which introduces it within the initial eight-week course, and there are specific programmes such as mindfulness-based compassionate living, where the compassion practices are central.

In our mindfulness for fatigue course, the calm abiding and insight practices are taught with implicit compassion. The intention is to pause and calm and then observe. People in the clinic often struggle to stop, and the protective system (nervous and immune systems) is observed as being in a state of constant work. Taking time to learn, to stop, soothe and calm has benefit on its own, but it is the insight that the friendly and compassionate pausing can offer that enables more fundamental changes to be made.

There are many texts and teachers teaching meditation in a detailed way, and studying and practising can be an interesting and rewarding endeavour personally. As practising clinicians, we do need to keep our practices alive but return to the course practices and maintain their integrity despite where our own practices may have taken us.

The mindfulness-based stress reduction (MBSR) (Santorelli et al. 2017) and mindfulness-based cognitive therapy (Segal et al. 2013) curriculums form the basis of this programme; the original MBSR course (Kabat-Zinn 2013) remains central, and the core intentions and practices in this mindfulness-based programme are fundamentally unchanged from this. Crane et al.'s (2021) *Essential Resources for Mindfulness Teachers* outlines the practices in detail, and Feldman and Kuyken's (2019) book *Mindfulness: Ancient Wisdom Meets Modern Psychology* is a detailed breakdown of mindfulness and its application in this context and format. *Mindfulness-Based Interventions: Teaching Assessment Criteria* (Kuyken et al. 2021) breaks down teaching into useful domains and is the basis of how we work.

These texts are amongst core trainings, and they highlight the reality that while each mindfulness-based course is specific to the teacher and the individuals, they do all follow a particular form. The courses follow the establishment of the four foundations of mindfulness (Crane 2017b; Feldman and Kuyken 2021):

- Mindfulness of the body
- Mindfulness of feeling tone (pleasant, unpleasant, neutral)
- Mindfulness of mind states
- Mindfulness of contents and processes of the mind.

The chapters in Part 2 are a description of what is taught on our course, with particular emphasis on elements of teaching that we have found to be of benefit to our participants.

Chapter 10

Practice Adaptations and Guidelines

- Sequence of practices through the course
- Particular teaching considerations
- Skills developed through the practices
- Structure of the practices

Many people we see are in a cycle of boom and bust, often really pushing themselves to complete tasks, socialize, etc., and then require a period of extended recovery. Stopping and pausing offers the opportunity to practise compassion and to reflect on what one has been doing and what may have contributed to the pushing into a 'boom'. Often, it is guilt or a desire to be as I always was and do things how I have always done them. People are learning mindfulness in our service with an understanding of the need to pace activity, manage baselines or limits on activity, prioritize, and deal with their all-or-nothing tendencies. Mindfulness is an opportunity to observe this while learning skills in stopping, calming and resting. People would not be in the clinic or on the mindfulness course if this was easy; the challenges in doing this are not perceived as obstacles, rather they are welcomed as the way in to a new way of living. In other words, obstacles *are* the path; the health condition and the challenges in managing it are what has brought us together, and finding ways through this is the whole point.

The invitation then is, as well as to learn *what* and *how* to practise, to work out *when* to practise and how to fold it into the day, using obstacles and challenges as part of the practice and supported by the group experience.

We will focus on what and how in the rest of this section and then consider how mindfulness participants fold into a day/week and use it to support their activity management and choices they make. This follows the structure of the course – we start off learning what mindfulness is; how it can be used to anchor and stop; consider what we notice when we can anchor and stop; and then become increasingly pragmatic and create a personal practice that informs and supports an active and participatory life grounded in the reality of each individual.

The main practices taught are the practices in mindfulness-based cognitive therapy (MBCT) and mindfulness-based stress reduction (MBSR) with some adaption:

- the body scan
- breath awareness
- three-step pause
- movement
- open awareness.

Each practice builds on the other and there is an emphasis on body awareness throughout, knowing and experiencing what is going on rather than thinking about experience. There are skills that are developed in the practices. They can be broken into:

- calming
- focused attention
- open monitoring
- compassionate acceptance
- insight and choices (including being aware of and developing resources).

Although they are presented in a sequence, each one supports the other and they are part of each other, for example we can't calm without making a choice to do so, and focused attention enables us to calm; insight leads us to choose an object of attention, and so on. Applying these skills to earthing or grounding and soothing self both during practice but also in daily life are explicitly taught early in the course.

Calming/grounding

There has been some debate about mindfulness not being relaxation; however, many find it relaxing, and there is benefit in being able to calm oneself and relax. Arguably, it is very hard to access wisdom and insight if one is wound up. Neurobiological understanding of trauma and distress suggests the brain is not able to learn when the amygdala is so strongly activated, and the ability to soothe enables the prefrontal cortex to 'come online' and optimize understanding, language and reason (Porges 2007; van der Kolk 2014). Contemporary Western teachers emphasize the soothing, calming nature of the practice and the role of challenging the constant busyness inherent in our culture (see e.g. Aylward 2021; Brach 2013).

A calming practice is initially introduced to help people stop, and can enable those with a background of trauma to manage. This starts with awareness of the environment through vision, sound and physical contact, letting the bodily system know where it is, taking the mind away from thinking towards inhabiting the current experience. Then to become aware of tension, holding and gripping, and actively using posture, breath and movement to let go of what can be let go of and letting be what remains. (This latter part is introducing wise action; we don't have to stay in the grip of tension, we can notice and make choices, but knowing that sometimes we may need to be with tension that cannot leave us and accept that the practice will not fix things instantly, if at all.)

Trauma-informed practice offers a practice that can be used when people start (and throughout the course). It is not particularly mindfulness, rather it supports creating the condition for mindfulness practice. It is based on working with fight/flight/freeze reactions that can be very hard to 'switch off' or even dial down, and then actively cultivating connection and soothing. It can be used before a practice, to relax, or before an activity, and seems to support people in resting as well as activity. The settling practice (outlined in the box) is an adaptation of Alastair Appleton's practices (see Resources section). We have made it gentler and easier to access for people with disabling health conditions. Feedback from patients is that this exercise can be very helpful as it includes movement and ways of thinking and encourages a compassionate stance. A guided version is available as part of the recordings for this course (see https://fionamckechnie.co.uk).

SETTLING PRACTICE

1. Look around the place you are – notice colours, shapes, textures – identify that there is nothing to fear here at the moment and say to yourself, 'Nothing to fear here right now.'
2. Bring your attention to sounds outside and inside the room and again say, 'Nothing to fear here right now.'
3. Feel where your body is in contact with the furniture, the floor, and so on. Put some pressure through your hands, feet, wherever you are in contact, so you can feel the surfaces; this is letting your body know where it is.
4. Take some deeper breaths, perhaps sighing and groaning on the out breath – phew! (as if in relief), and look around again saying, 'Nothing to fear here right now.'
5. Bring your attention to your arms (the limbs of 'fight'), your shoulders and neck, make some circular movements, shrug and let the movement move down your arms, making circular movements with your elbows, forearms, wrists and hands. Make the

movements free-form and don't attempt to be symmetrical, the arms and fists are how we fight, we cannot fight if we are making circular shapes; make starfish shapes with your hands, again don't try hard and don't stretch. Perhaps shake out and say, 'Nothing to fight here.'

6. Come to your jaw (another way we fight), waggle your jaw, make sounds, sigh, groan and say, 'Nothing to fight here.'

7. Breathe and sigh. Feel your belly move with the breath and reassure yourself, 'Nothing to fear or fight here.'

8. Come to your feet and legs (limbs of 'flight') and press through your heels (we run on our toes, so activating heels means we can't run) and say, 'Nothing to flee here.'

9. Make circles with your toes and ankles and let the movement go through your legs, with random, circular-type movements; let them shake and say, 'Nothing to flee here.'

10. Come to a stillness if you can; otherwise, let the body move, shake, etc. as it wishes, no need to control things.

11. Sighing breath: 'Nothing to fear here.'

12. Come to your belly and place your hands on your diaphragm, and if it feels OK, take some deep breaths and say, 'Nothing to fear here.'

13. Come to your face and make a few big cheesy grins (muscles of connection). 'It's OK.'

14. Sigh, move as feels good.

15. Come to your eyes (muscles of connection), and while keeping your head still, take both eyes in one direction as far as they can; when they want to come back (strong urge, perhaps with a yawn, a sigh, a burp) let them come back and go again the same side then the other. 'It's OK.'

16. Gently allow the body to rest; if you need to move do so; if you wish to sleep, roll over and sleep; if you wish to do something, do it, taking your calmness with you – 'Nothing to fear here, right now. It's OK.'

Sleepiness and relaxation

One adaptation we perhaps make is to be very relaxed about sleepiness and falling asleep. Many of our participants have huge difficulties with sleep and rest, and part of the self-management approach is to explore the continuum between low-level activity, rest and sleep, so giving space to explore what this feels like is useful.

If someone reports that they have fallen asleep, this can be a significant improvement in their quality of life and can lead to practices that support sleep. The challenge is, that we *fall* asleep, and what may have helped the sleep is the non-goal-directed nature of the practice; doing it with no expectation can lead to an increase in well-being as expectation and tension are released. This then becomes the focus of inquiry, and gentle curiosity can help explore what 'worked'.

The same process occurs with an experience of relaxation, which can be enormously helpful to someone who lives with chronic pain and fatigue. But there is a nuanced edge between, on the one hand, becoming relaxed while practising and, on the other, being able to gently self-regulate and take care of oneself when feeling stressed and using a practice intentionally to relax. Rather, we need to explore what it feels like to do this, and meet with equanimity, relaxation and tension in the practice and within the group inquiry. Eliciting experiences of tension, awkwardness, frustration and being equally curious and supportive of that as a valid experience can help this process. As we go forward with the group, it is the turning towards experience, being curious and kind, having patience and trusting the non-doing that can lead to experiences of well-being. But somehow holding this lightly...

Focused attention

Being able to pay attention stabilizes the mind and forms the basis of the other skills. Being able to stop and pause with intention is the basis of anchoring and pausing. This then enables insights to emerge and develops a meta-awareness of the workings of the mind, our habits and patterns. It is important at the start to emphasize the difference between concentration and attention. People with pain and fatigue will report periods of brain fog, where their concentration and ability to focus are significantly affected. This point is emphasized in Session 2, when people often report feeling like a failure because they fell asleep, their mind wandered away from the guided practice, and so on. The inquiry draws out that mindfulness is about noticing *all* of that and that choosing to come back *is* the practice (Figures 10.1 and 10.2). Asking about how it felt when they return to the guidance or what they are using as an object of attention helps clarify this. Also discussing that this is a different way to learn, the skill we are developing is the noticing and choosing rather than the doing or getting it right. The following quotes are reported examples of what it feels like to notice mind wandering rather than trying to stop it.

> 'It was a huge relief when you told me I didn't need to listen to everything or even follow all the guidance. Working with the guidance and acknowledging where I was and being curious about it was novel and at times fun.'

'It wasn't until after the third session that I really understood what being non-judgemental and gentle with myself meant. It didn't matter that my thoughts drifted off during the exercises. All I needed to do was to be aware that they had and gently bring myself back to focusing on my breathing. That was what being mindful was about.'

What we think we are doing when we practise mindfulness

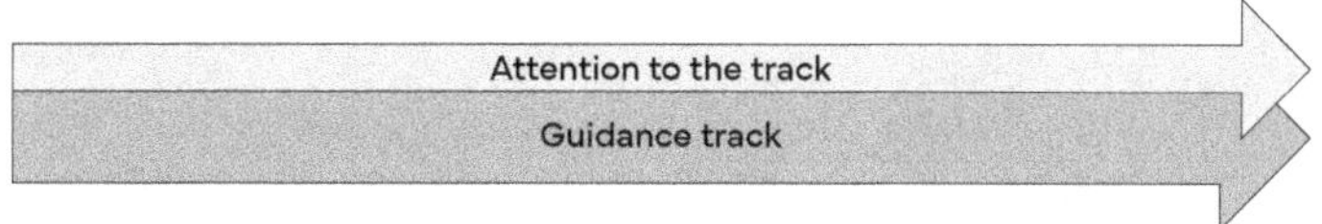

What we are actually doing when we practise mindfulness

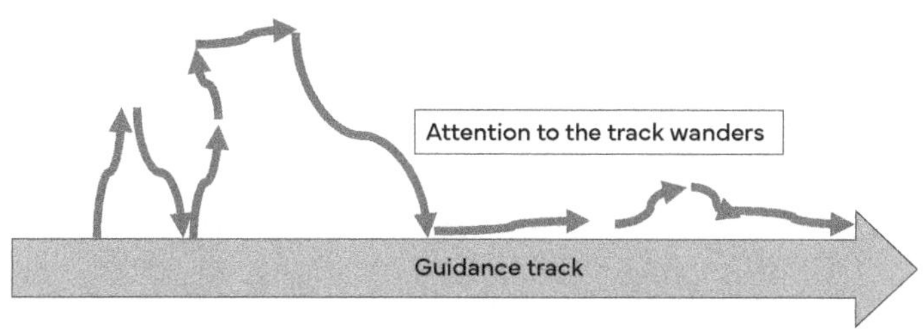

Figure 10.1 What we think we are doing when we practise mindfulness vs. what we are actually doing

Good news is that mindfulness choice is noticing that the mind is wandering all over the place, falling asleep or listening to the track

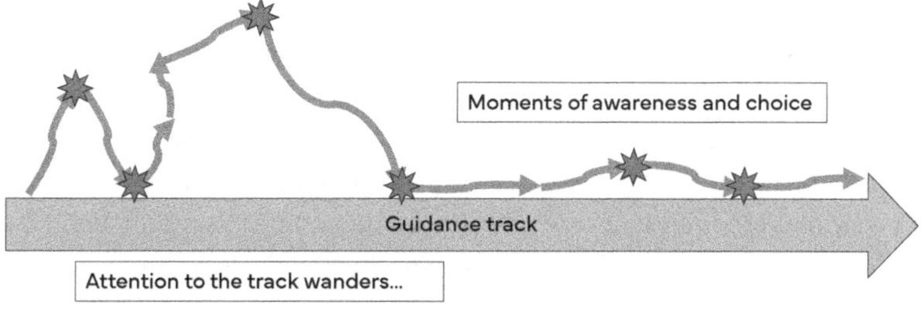

Figure 10.2 Mindfulness is awareness of mind wandering as much as staying on the track

Choosing an object of attention is a practice of itself. Objects of attention can be very tangible or subtle (based on Pollak et al. 2014). This is not hierarchical, there is no target of moving from the very tangible to the very subtle, the emphasis is on making wise choices about what is needed now (Table 10.1). This is not a concentration practice, it is awareness, and if we cannot pay attention, then that is information, and our practice is to notice that we are repeatedly drawn to different components of our experience and to remain curious about that.

Table 10.1 Objects of attention (adapted from Pollak et al. 2014)

Tangible	Movement/walking, etc.	Grounding/calming – can be helpful to stabilize when distracted or when arousal state is high, cannot assume where a sense of grounding might be. Guide choice and experimentation with different points
↑	Feet touching ground	
	Sights and sounds	
	Contact with the chair/floor, etc.	'Where do you feel sense of safety, or can be anchored right now?'
	Taste/eating	
	Hands and fingers	
	Breath in the belly	The breath and the more subtle sensation in the body can be objects of attention when we are less agitated
	Air at tip of the nose	
	Sense of space in the centre of the body	
↓	Thoughts – experienced as a sense, e.g. like sounds	
Subtle	Emotions – felt sense	How do you know you are joyful, sad, etc.? Where and how is this experienced somatically?

Open monitoring

Rather than having a particular object of focus, we bring awareness to what is going on in the present moment. This requires us to cultivate curiosity and acceptance, noting what we like, what we don't like, what we would normally miss or ignore. This often raises paradoxes of being in pain and being relaxed at the same time; of feeling sad, yet also pleased about something else; that while I may feel terrible right now, there are other things happening and that this mood and feeling can change very much in the way the weather can change. The recognition that thoughts are just thoughts and that beliefs are just beliefs, not necessarily facts or absolute truths, despite the seed of truth that sparks the thinking, can be liberating as we have insights into the nature of our own and others' suffering and the option to make choices.

For example, when my children were younger and fought, I noticed I clenched my jaw, felt a heaviness in my body and tension in my shoulders and then often found myself eating crunchy things, which quite often were biscuits... I would have liked to resist the biscuits, but what happened was this awareness led me to choose to relax my jaw and shoulders, look around and take a break that may or may not have involved biscuits, and I generally felt less tense and stressed and could address my catastrophic thinking and worries that I was a total failure at raising children; then I could take steps to manage the kids but from a more relaxed position. If I had made it about reducing my biscuit eating, I would have had something else to worry about, which would have probably increased the tension and most likely have led to further biscuit eating and more negative thoughts.

In the clinic, individuals have found that they have identified particularly intense symptoms, such as pain, digestion problems and heaviness in the limbs, and have been able to work with the tension they have surrounding it, both mentally and physically. We have multiple instances of people reporting that their pain is not everywhere as they thought, but is in a constant state of flux and that their reactions may change depending on other factors, for example when they have overdone things, are pushing or are cross or frightened of their symptoms and want to 'win':

> 'Mindfulness has completely changed how I manage my CFS/ME. It helps me to more fully recognize my symptoms, instead of ignore or block them. When I recognize them, then I can work on dealing with them. I am actively working on accepting the symptoms. I am more aware of the signs that indicate I am heading towards a crisis. I have learnt how and what to do when I recognize stress.'

> 'It's allowed me to feel a bit more in control of my body, mind and general well-being. I feel that it keeps bad mental health at bay and reminds me of the bigger picture. It's helped me understand and be aware of different sensations in my body which had allowed me to communicate more precisely and accurately with my doctors regarding pain (prickly, tingling, sharp, dull, etc.). It helps them do their job and means I get more accurate and quicker help.'

Compassionate acceptance

The cultivation of compassion is taught on some mindfulness courses as discrete practices; for example, creating an image of a compassionate other, a compassionate colour, etc. In mindfulness-based cognitive therapy, it is not taught *per se*, rather it is implicit within the practice and how the therapy is delivered. It could be useful to develop this in a later course, and a compassionate approach is part of mindfulness. The practices cannot be taught without a friendly open awareness (Segal et al. 2013, chapter 8).

> The quality of mindfulness is not a neutral or blank presence. True mindfulness is imbued with warmth, compassion, and interest. In the light of this engaged attention we discover it is impossible to hate or fear anything...that we truly understand. The nature of mindfulness is engagement: where there is interest, a natural unforced attention follows. (Christina Feldman, quoted in Segal et al. 2013, pp.137–8)

This warm and compassionate approach to our experience is perhaps where the transformation lies, and ultimately this is how we relate to ourselves. The relational aspect of this is explicitly broken down in the second domain of the mindfulness-based interventions teaching assessment criteria (Kuyken et al. 2021). Five key features are considered in this domain, which are presented as being about how clinicians are with the group participants. However, it could perhaps be used to consider how we relate to ourselves and our experience of symptoms, stress and their consequences and how this intrapersonal relationship can be supported by mindfulness. These key features are:

- Authenticity and potency – relating in a way which seems genuine, honest and confident
- Connection and acceptance – actively attending to and connecting with participants and their present-moment experience and conveying back an accurate and empathic understanding of this
- Compassion and warmth – conveying a deep awareness, sensitivity, appreciation and openness to participants' experience
- Curiosity and respect – conveying genuine interest in each participant and his/her experience while respecting each participant's vulnerabilities, boundaries and need for privacy
- Mutuality – engaging with the participants in a mutual and collaborative working relationship.

In the group mindfulness sessions the leaders offer these qualities initially to participants who can both experience a compassionate way of relating personally during conversations; but there is a mutuality when we witness others engaging compassionately with people's struggles with the practices. They then in turn can offer this to each other in small groups and dyads and ultimately to themselves. It is possible to see that compassion arises or emerges from the mindfulness practice (both the guided practices and the practice of listening and being with others and sharing) and that allows new ways of acting and being.

A compassionate shift showed up in our interviews with participants in response to the question: 'How has mindfulness helped you manage your health condition?'

'I'm more patient and kind to myself.'

'It's hugely increased my self-awareness so I'm better placed to understand my habits and patterns, and why/when they're getting me into trouble; and allowing me to focus my practice on those areas likely to be of most benefit. It's helpful for pacing and taking more appropriate and timely action. The most significant benefit has been in increasing my self-compassion, and the many knock-on benefits that has.'

'In every way, to breathe with mindfulness enables me to put things into perspective, which in turn enables me to approach the challenging dilemmas of the everyday in a calm and collected way, to respond with a calm reason and authoritative self-assurance.'

'I am less angry and impatient, so able to enjoy those simple little things in my daily life. Sometimes I am overwhelmed at how many good things happen in a day, when in the past, I wouldn't have recognized good events, even when they were really obvious.'

'I am so much kinder towards myself. More compassionate towards others and less judgemental on myself and others. Maybe I am not such a perfectionist, and that is a relief, as it took a lot of energy to maintain such high standards.'

Insight and wise choices

While the practice invites us to pause and notice, the group inquiry enables people to hear how others are managing and what changes they are making. To raise awareness of personal resources, as well as asking what they experienced, we may go on to ask about how people managed. For example, someone who had felt nauseous during a practice: 'I opened my eyes, looked around, changed my posture and found a way back into the practice at my own pace.' At the beginning of a session and each practice, we invite people to check in with how they are now, acknowledge what they have been doing, and inquire into what their body needs. For some this is novel as they are so used to pushing through. For example, a nurse reflected that they often don't even know when they need to use the toilet; some people acknowledge they are thirsty; others that they need to stretch or lie down.

We give space and time for people to acknowledge not only how they are but also what they might need to do about it, and to consider how much energy they need to put into the session, bearing in mind the rest of their day. This has become more important since we have a switched to online delivery during the pandemic, when some were squeezing the session into work and family life rather than taking time out to come to a space where they would be undisturbed and also being unavailable during the travel time. The online delivery has meant there are opportunities for people to use what is in their own environment to help themselves, and we suspect there is more carry-over into daily life. When we run in-room sessions we have a variety of blankets, cushions, different types of chairs, a variety of teas, and so on, and often participants would get things for each other and help each other out. The online scenario means there is more self-sufficiency, but perhaps that has increased the carry-over into daily life?

The question 'How do I need to work now?' can inform how the practice is done; do I do it in a relaxed way going underneath what is being said and phase in and out? Or do I take measures to be alert? For example, by staying sat up rather than lying down or by holding up a hand when doing a body scan to let me know when I have fallen asleep, etc. We hope to model that both ways are appropriate, and it is part of the intention and choice component of the practice. There is also the invitation to change; for example, if someone is sitting and then they realize they need to lie down. If there is uncertainty, then inviting people to set themselves up for both and to make the transition according to what is needed. This is to disrupt the tendency that many people we see have to all-or-nothing thinking and behaviour and living by strict rules. We widen this out to attendance and encourage people to come to the session even if they are late. In online sessions, there is no compulsion to turn the camera on.

The following are quotes from participants reflecting on participating in the group in a way that they could manage at that point, and on the impact that has had on their wider self-management:

> 'I've never done that before, come in late to anything. It felt OK, actually it felt good, I was welcomed and it made me realize I'm doing the best I can.'

> 'I came [to a Zoom session] sure I wouldn't put my camera on, but by the end I felt better and was able to join in; it surprised me as I thought online work made me more tired.'

At the end of a practice the invitation to take a wise and compassionate choice for oneself is repeated: 'What do I need to do now to take care of myself?' One participant reflected that she has that as a refrain throughout her day and has found she has been able to do more as she will alter things so they are achievable.

Structure of a mindfulness practice

Therapists leading the practice do so from their own experience of the practice in the moment. This skill needs to be developed as part of supervision and training, and the therapists need to have experience of both the practice and the stage of the group. Using a script is not appropriate, the words need to flow from the practice. It is recommended that therapists listen to a wide variety of practices, preferably work with a teacher and a system for a sustained period of time and go on retreats developing their own authentic style while returning to the basics of the practice on the course.

Table 10.2 is based on notes given to people in Session 5 to practise without a guidance track and is the basis for all the practices and how we have been teaching within the course.

Table 10.2 Basic structure for all the guided practices

Features of the practice	Notes/rationale
Your intention • What do you intend to do? • How long for? Maybe use a timer.	Being explicit about both what the practice will involve and how long it will be can enable them to make choices about posture, props, etc.
Physical setup • Place preferably not disturbed (if at all possible!). • Choose posture and props you might need.	In a Zoom group this may mean people move away from the screen or perhaps they can't get into an ideal position and hear you, balancing out the need for comfort and engagement. In the room we might need to help people with props and position, model posture, support, etc. Encourage 'do what you need to do to take care of yourself' – this is part of the implicit compassionate approach. A short practice at the start of the session can help people tune in to where they are today and make adaptations with posture, props, etc. from how they are now.
Arrival/landing • Allow your body to land into the posture you have chosen, take time to allow movements, wriggles, feel the contact with the floor, chair, etc. • Notice what you can see, hear – drop into sensory experience rather than naming, judging (e.g. colour, shape, volume, tone). • Notice any additional bracing or tensing in the body and invite it to soften. • Scan through the body briefly allowing any parts to move, soften, etc.	This is an important part of the practice and is an essential part of a trauma-informed approach – helping people unwind or unlock from tension and find points of stability. In the first few sessions it is important to spend time on this because, whether they are in an actual room or a virtual room, they are among strangers doing a strange thing. This part of the practice can also be done during activity or when someone notices they are becoming dysregulated. It introduces 'coming to the body' to stabilize and soothe and taking care of the physical rather than having to talk oneself into feeling better. People can shift and breathe and use their environment to feel better.

cont.

Features of the practice	Notes/rationale
Acknowledgement • Take stock of how you are right now – thoughts, feelings, sensations – spend time on this, allowing opening. Your body may need to shift; allow this. • Find your feet; explore your contact with the surface you are on. • Find your way into an open, upright or (gently lengthened) dignified posture; finding alignment from the inside. • Let your mind settle on the movements of the breath. • Check in with intention; how do you need to practise?	This is part of arriving, and again is worth spending time on; acknowledging how we are encourages wise choices rather than doing what we habitually do, or in this context what someone might think the therapist is telling them to do. People are also consciously using posture to find physical and mental alignment, creating a container for where they will be placing their attention. This encourages embodied attention and an awareness that shifts are not just mental experiences and that the mind inhabits the whole body and is affected by it and that attention can affect the whole system. Asking how we need to practise is useful and again encourages innate wisdom: 'Do I need to rest and be gentle, perhaps letting the words wash over me, or do I want a crisp attention to the practice? Or somewhere in-between?' The metaphor of a stringed instrument is useful – if it's too tight it won't play well, but neither will it if it is too loose. This can change day by day.
Main practice • Could be a focused-attention body scan, mindfulness of breathing, sounds or thoughts. • Or you can sit and breathe, and when your experience shifts to being very aware of sounds or sensations, become mindful of sounds or sensations, then return to the breath, and so on.	Whether it is a focused practice or open monitoring, the practice is compassionate, steeped in the values of patience, curiosity, trust, acceptance, non-judging, non-striving and letting go (the attitudinal foundations of mindfulness, in *Full Catastrophe Living* by Jon Kabat-Zinn) See session plans and Kuyken et al. 2021, Domain 4, for details of each practice.
Attitude ♥ Practise kindness, patience, acceptance, trust, curiosity every time you return to your intended practice; every time the mind wanders off; when you realize you are impatient, judgemental, have fallen asleep…	This underpins all that we are doing; wisdom and choices need to come from a place of compassion, not self-improvement. There is a discipline to this, it is not 'anything goes', as the nature of the mind is often to wander and we also habitually self-criticize. Practising kindness can be novel, challenging and unnerving.
Finishing Appreciate yourself for what you have done; what do you need now? How can you take the practice into the rest of your day?	This 'seals' the practice and explicitly directs attention to what's next, enabling the possibility of using mindfulness throughout the day. In Buddhist traditions, it is common to send wishes of kindness to others, acknowledging that while we do the practice for ourselves, it is also of benefit to others.

Specific considerations on the use of MBCT and MBSR practices

The body scan

As with many mindfulness courses, this is the first practice we teach, and there are no particular adaptations beyond what is described in Table 10.2, and people are given choices of 15- and 30-minute practices. We emphasize choice to undermine all-or-nothing approaches and to offer a graded method consistent with the self-management approach used across the team. Better to start small and regular, rather than occasionally do something to a fuller extent but less often.

Awareness practice

This is often called a 'sitting practice' in both MBCT and MBSR; we have chosen to call it 'awareness' to encourage people to spend time considering how they wish to practise today and being in an appropriate posture. This builds with short practices scattered through the course. The short practices feed each other and the longer practices; like a necklace they are similar and linked. Shorter pauses are used throughout the programme and are perhaps the most powerful and potent element, particularly the ability to 'come to the body'. The short practices include:

- *Vision* – Taking in what I can see in my environment, acknowledging where I am, noticing exits and then dropping beneath language and noticing colour, shape, texture, quality of light; shapes within shapes; colours within colours.
- *Sound*   Placing attention on sounds, dropping beneath the name of the sound and experiencing the pitch, volume, direction. Noticing the direction of the sound, sounds in the distance, sounds up close. Feeling the sound with the whole body. Noticing spaces between sounds, silence around the sounds... Sounds within sounds, changing nature of sound.
- *Finding my feet* – Placing attention on feet; feeling the ground, weight dropping; centre of gravity lowering; spine rising; shoulders rolling back; allowing movement throughout the body; deeper breaths... Taking care of myself.
- *Anchoring* – Doing 'vision' and 'finding my feet' practices, then becoming aware of the whole body and scanning through my body and environment noticing what is pleasant or soothing, or somewhere I want to rest; somewhere I can anchor right now and then letting the mind wander and gently return to the anchor; becoming absorbed in the anchor.

EMBODIED PAUSE
(i.e. using the body to stop, pause and regroup)

This can be particularly useful if we have mental fatigue or have a lot of thoughts going around. Rather than having to think our way into stopping, we can use our body; it can be done in ten seconds or ten minutes or longer:

- Find your feet (focus as far away from your head as possible!).
- Feel into the surface you are sitting, standing or lying on.
- Let the furniture and floor take your weight.
- Give in to gravity – you might slump or flop, that's OK – give up for a moment.
- Sigh, yawn, groan.
- Realign by slowly starting with feet come into an upright posture with a sense of up lift through the back and the neck, gently supporting the head.
- Lift through the chest, so there is space between the pelvis and the sternum.
- Keep your attention on where you are in touch with the floor – image of a mountain or a tree can be helpful – rising up tall yet rooted.
- Soften hands, face, belly.
- Breathe.
- What do you need to do next?
- Make a plan based on what arises.

Additional eye movements
In the relaxed upright posture or aligned lying posture:

- Look around your space taking in colours, textures, light, etc., then come to stillness.
- Keep the head still.
- Move the eyes in one direction as far as they can go and hold.
- When you get the urge, come back to centre, possibly accompanied by a yawn, sigh, burp.
- Repeat same side, then twice other side.
- Then do the same again but look to the side and downwards.

Three-step pause

This practice was adapted from the MBCT three-minute breathing space to have more emphasis on pausing and resting and to use any anchor, not just the breath as the focused awareness. While we did this as part of the course, in response to a number of participants being unable to focus on the centre of the body, and our intention to encourage wise choice and psychological flexibility rather than follow specific rules, this was in line with general adaptations initially from the work done in trauma-informed mindfulness (Crane et al. 2021; Treleaven 2018) but also in response to Covid-19, which affected breathing and increased general levels of anxiety throughout the population.

It follows the breathing space hour glass and can be done in a minute, three minutes, 15 minutes or half an hour. This is actually a complex practice despite the seemingly simple name and the short length. It is arguably the most important practice as it incorporates so much of the course and then integrates into a workable and practical practice that can be used throughout the day. The full form is taught towards the end of the course.

THREE-STEP PAUSE

Step 1: What is here?

Awareness of environment, thoughts, feelings; sensations, posture – not changing, stopping and noticing – the questions 'What's up for me right now?' or 'What's the internal weather like now?' can help bring a gentle curiosity to the moment. Recalling that we are interested explorers rather than a SWAT team trying to eradicate annoyances and challenges. This becomes more developed after Session 5.

Step 2: Gentle attention

Gathering the body into posture for attention, starting with grounding through the felt sense and contact with chair (if sitting, etc.), scanning the current experience (environment, body, etc.) and finding an anchor, maintaining attention in the anchor through gentle absorption, letting the mind wander then find its way back.

Step 3: Expanding

Feeling into the whole body, moving if wished; feeling in the earth; vision; sound. Asking: What do I need to do now to take care of myself and this moment?

Teaching consideration: Mind-wandering and anchoring

After much experimentation, practice, reflection and supervision (thanks to my supervisor Taravajra for long detailed discussions on this), we have been taking a particular approach to mind-wandering in the interests of encouraging an attitude of 'allowing' and reducing tension. Instead of saying 'when the mind wanders gently bring it back', we have been inviting the mind to wander *after* spending time on developing an anchor. This is designed to undercut the idea that mind-wandering is 'wrong' and to be worked with; it happens, but when it does, we notice there are choices rather than something to be 'improved'.

Practising letting the mind wander and then letting it find its way back to the anchor explicitly identifies that there is a part of us that can do this, that can see what is going on and make choices. This in turn develops the anchor – 'How do you feel when you return to the anchor?' 'What's it like to return?'

In later sessions we can add in more choice: 'When you notice the wandering mind, what's that like?' and 'What do you want to do? Continue on a train of thought, in a memory or whatever, or do you wish to return to the anchor?'

Later still: 'Notice the mind wandering, and consider your intention for this practice, is this still appropriate? What do you wish to do with your attention?'

This process is based on understanding of the challenge of cognitive fatigue (see chapter 7). We know that many people struggle to attend and concentrate to the extent that they struggle to read, find words, manage conversation or be in places with multiple sensory demands. How the practice described above works with brain fog is first by resourcing oneself through the body, easing out tension, and the brain is released from the job of being on high alert. If in settling one is aware of being tense and 'foggy', then the practice can stay there, soothing, perhaps moving, doing things that are known to help – connecting with nature or perhaps resting, and so on. It is crucial to back off from pushing the brain to work any harder than it already is. This is because we know (from work in neurology and brain injury) that a stressed brain cannot improve cognitive performance. One must go at the brain's pace.

Dealing with challenges and being-with-difficulty practice

Turning towards difficulty, learning to respond rather than react is why people come to the courses. This process is seeded early and unfolds through the course, and each participant will have their own experience and capacity to turn towards difficulty. As already discussed, the challenge participants face is not only living with the condition, but living with the changes and adaptations one has to make to manage it, or live well with fatigue and pain. The fluctuating nature of the condition means that the capacity to manage can vary hugely.

The practice of managing challenges or difficult times builds on the previous work: there is a settling or grounding actively using the body – dropping and then rebuilding or constructing an upright or aligned posture that enables some gentle focus. This leads to a check-in or appraisal of state of mind – spacious, jumpy, zoned out, etc. – and a gentle focus that can support attending to the present moment and be of itself soothing. We have built the practices over a few weeks, particularly finding resources within the body that are accessible in the present moment, and acknowledged pleasant and unpleasant experiences and a sense of the changing nature of experience; akin to the weather it can change for all sorts of unseen reasons moment by moment. Working directly with challenge as a focus for the practice can seem counterintuitive (as the focus on unpleasant experience in Session 4 may too). The following quotes are typical reflections after this practice:

> 'I feel more rested'; 'My heart rate reduced for the first time in weeks'; 'It changes'; 'I can drop the fight'; 'I can do more with this than I thought'; 'It's very relaxing.'

We start off with a simple exercise to look at responses to difficulty; in a room session we used finger traps to demonstrate the movement of coming towards to make space and then carefully extracting the finger, which is in direct opposition to the intuitive reaction that we must pull away. On Zoom sessions we have a YouTube clip from *Star Trek* of Data getting stuck in a finger trap. This makes the same point, and normally a few people have come across the finger traps and explain how they feel when 'stuck' in one and the way out.

In the practice we consider the reaction to pull away but give examples of ways of gently turning towards difficulty and emphasizing the importance of going at one's own pace:

1. Simply saying 'this is difficult' and redirecting attention to something more soothing.
2. Doing 1, then acknowledging where the difficulty is felt in the body – its general location, then its more precise location, its shape, depth, colour perhaps, texture. Exploring it like a botanist rather than a weed controller or, as Segal et al. (2013) say, 'on the work bench of the mind'. Coming away and soothing as much as required.
3. Then using a sweeping attention in time with the breath, 'breathe into the area of difficulty'.
4. Coming to the whole body, dropping and settling again, and choosing a point of focus.
5. Being aware of this moment, sensations, thoughts, feelings, quality of the mind.

6. Becoming aware of any difficulty arising. If it is the same difficulty, being aware of how it is now. There can be a deepening and softening if we need to return to a familiar feeling or pattern of reactivity and start at 1 again – choosing to acknowledge or explore as feels appropriate in this moment.

Points to be aware of: because we have developed soothing and grounding in the earlier practices, perhaps resulting in a feeling of well-being, there can be a tendency to feel as though one *should* be able to cope, or there can be an experience that the difficulty is shut off quickly, which can feel gratifying. Trying to cope can become a form of disconnect or 'bypassing' where the practice is used to dam up difficult feelings; then if they arise, that is because the person is 'not doing it right'. This is the Doing mode at work, trying to fix and improve, to solve the problem through the practice.

To clarify then – we use the grounding and develop skills in soothing to allow the difficulty to be present, to allow an exploration in a way that feels doable, and in the first instance to take care of ourselves and then to allow the feelings to be present and turning towards them *with no intention other than to be curious* – we are *not* trying to get rid or manage them. This intention is crucial to build up a 'Being mind' attitude. We can then be curious about what unfolds, what happens when we allow and gently investigate the nooks and crannies of difficulty, be it a pain, a tension, a knot of anxiety: What tells us we feel like this? What precisely are we labelling? Where is it?

Example of being-with-difficulty practice

I have had a difficult piece of information arrive as a text message. I notice I feel stressed and anxious. I know I need to work out how to respond skilfully. I pause, feel my feet on the floor, notice I want to run and my palms feel sweaty, my mouth is dry and my stomach clenches.

In order to counteract the fight/flight, I work with the limbs that will fight or run, so I purposely move my feet and wrist in circles and let my body shake. I acknowledge this is a challenging and painful time and feel the contact my body is making with the chair, let my weight go down to the earth and feel the support of the earth. I give in to holding it altogether and stop trying to cope.

(If I stayed here, I may feel OK, but I am passive and the problem is not addressed and soon enough it may come back. And actually if I stay here, I am immobile and may resort to other activity to keep me numbed out.)

Then I regroup, or rebuild my self through the body, rising up through the spine, keeping my feet on the floor, using the image of a tree or mountain to feel both rooted yet tall and have a sense of substance that rises up. I feel into both a sense of uplift rising from the pelvis and up into the chest and the sense of space this creates. I become aware of the movement my breath is making in the body, placing attention on movement at the back and the belly. This is creating space. I haven't got rid of anything, but I am aware of strength, alignment, and then focusing on my anchor (the breath) I can experience each moment and be in the present. I then look at the text again, breathe and allow myself to feel the confusion and anxiety. I go to where it hurts – a tension in my heart, a feeling of nausea, tight jaw – and explore it whilst keeping a wider sense of the body, its strength and capacity to be in the moment. I breathe in and out of my heart, placing a hand on my chest. This is tender, painful. I feel sadness and am aware of a tear. I also touch into what I care about, what I understand, my beliefs about the situation. My response to the message needs to come from my beliefs and values, not my pain and anxiety.

How can I take care of myself? Acknowledge this is hard, then look for what is OK right now. What information do I need to respond? Where can I get some help?

I haven't changed the content of the message (or the sender's beliefs) but I have been able to access a more responsive place, acknowledge what I can change by taking care of myself and respond in line with how I wish to behave. I can move on, leaving what cannot be changed. Aware there is a chink of pain remaining, but this is not overwhelming; if anything it reminds me to go gently and be aware I may need to take this into account in other interactions throughout the day. I return to the grounding practice throughout the day and move with stretches and walking and continue to scan through for difficulties, allowing and nurturing them as I go. Then send my reply once I have had a chance to consider my options.

Body, mind and action are one cohesive whole – a difficulty arises and most of the system reacts to fight it or run away, which, if not a simple problem, will compound the challenge. The response mode allows us to see outside of our situation and find resources that are both internal and external. It may mean asking for help or comfort from someone else, but it also allows us to access internal resources within the body/mind/action. The difficulty does not go away, but perhaps it is more workable.

CASE EXAMPLES

Jemima used this practice and reported that she felt supported by being able to access the body; she had had a burglary earlier in the year so, as well as managing ME/CFS, felt she had prolonged stress and a very reactive anxiety reaction. Working directly with the physical sensation meant there was something she could do about how she was feeling. Being able to gently turn towards what was there meant she could start to tenderly identify her reactions. By the end of the course she felt there were was much to continue to learn and develop through this practice.

Anthea, who lives with fibromyalgia and has significant levels of pain, reported that she has an entirely different relationship with pain now; she no longer sees it as something to be fought. She used the body scan to turn towards what was present, feeling that staying there for a while, exploring what she felt, meant it gave her a chance to acknowledge and not fight it. She found the structure of the body scan helpful as it meant the practice would move around the body and she had more appreciation for the areas of her body that were OK, in fact more than OK that she could enjoy them. She also identified that previously her pain had driven her to try harder, and now she was better able to plan and pace herself rather than push and come from a place of 'driven doing' or reactive stress. She was intrigued that her family (whom she communicated with via Zoom as they were in Lagos) could see that she was feeling better and had asked her about her 'new medication'.

SUMMARY

- The adaptations are targeted at soothing the dysregulated protective system (see Part 1). There is an emphasis on a graded approach – start small and build up and emphasize grounding and soothing in the first instance followed by asking 'How can I take care of myself in this moment?'
- Compassion practices are not actively taught; however, the practices and inquiry are imbued with compassion and the cultivation of wise self-care.
- Working actively with fight/flight/freeze can help people unwind.
- Sleepiness can be optimized to support better sleep and rest.
- Brain fog can disrupt practices; understanding this means participants can go with it and work at their own brain's pace. Reducing stress is crucial to managing cognitive problems.

Chapter 11

Developing Awareness Through Inquiry

WE CAN BECOME AWARE – SO WHAT?

- Using inquiring questions to develop insight
- How awareness and insight are developed over the course
- Experiential learning and the group
- Embodied understanding
- Challenges and benefits of awareness

Developing insight

Inquiry can perhaps be framed as: Asking questions that increase perception and engagement with what we are experiencing, leading to opportunities for change.

After each practice is an inquiry into what happened. This questioning after a practice is an intrinsic part of the practice and can be regarded as a practice itself. It can be used in the mindful awareness of daily activity as much as in a formal practice. The questions in the session hopefully generate a kindly curiosity about what is happening and thereby lead to more choice points or options as to a way forward. As mindfulness cultivates awareness, opportunities for insight arise that may change our understanding and open us up to other ways of thinking and doing.

By verbalizing what has been experienced directly, we can reinforce and nuance understanding cognitively. Often, it is not until someone talks through what happens that they realize what has happened and make sense of it. This creates the possibility for what Shapiro et al. (2006) term 're-perceiving'. Rhonda Knight's description of her reappraisal of her situation during her first mindfulness course is an example of this:

My main conclusion from completing the positive event diary and reflecting on it in the session was that I don't *have* to have family close to hand to be cared for when feeling unwell. That profound insight into my support network here in the UK helped me to feel not so scared and alone in my struggle to live with the symptoms of ME/CFS. Compared to the start of the week, my perspective on life was beginning to change...

An approach rather than a set of techniques

Mindfulness practices are best thought of as a way of being rather than a collection of techniques (Kabat-Zinn et al. 2013). They are all ways that point to a way of being with our world rather than as tools to solve particular problems or access particular ways of being. The attitudes and relationship to our experiences we are cultivating are just as important as the specific techniques. In other words, the recordings and guidance we use are literally *practice* for how to be in your actual life. One may experience happiness, relaxation and peacefulness, and appreciate and enjoy those in your practice, then notice them more vividly in day-to-day life. This also works the other way, an experience in daily life that we identify as being the result of the practice, for example increased awareness of nature, a moment of calm or responsiveness rather than reacting, can reinforce the benefits of the daily 'exercise' of formal practice. In this way, the inquiry can form a bridge from the experiences in the formal practice into day-to-day activities or vice versa (Figure 11.1).

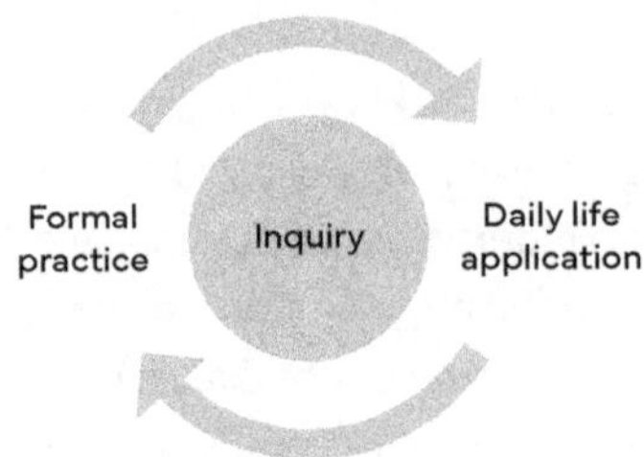

Figure 11.1 Formal practice and daily life application support each other

Awareness

In order to inquire we need awareness for its own sake. Managing the human tendency to not problem solve or fix anyone is key to the approach. Awareness enables insight, which in turn enables choice, which of itself increases self-management of challenging situations.

All mindfulness-based programmes are designed to enhance life by not only managing the unwanted components of existence, but actively 'turning towards' them. For all of us, 'being more aware' can be confusing, contradictory and stressful, as well as useful, supportive and fruitful.

Mindful awareness has an implicit compassion and empathy, and it is more than 'reporting' what is here, which indeed can be a pitfall where one is very observant of what the internal and emotional process is, but unable to let go to and access rest and compassion. This warm, empathic awareness fosters wisdom, enabling the possibility of living in almost an entirely different way, based on the reality and choices available now, rendering a mindfulness-based approach helpful and supportive in day-to-day life.

How awareness and attention are developed during the programme

There is a movement from the basis of 'paying attention' in the present moment to a broader awareness over time of resources, patterns and habits:

- Awareness – what am I aware of now – five senses and thinking, internal and external
- Curiosity, acceptance, friendliness to what I am aware of
- Awareness of pleasant/unpleasant, i.e. I like some things but don't like others
- Noting thoughts, feelings and behaviours in response to how I am feeling (elaborating on pleasant/unpleasant)
- Becoming aware of resources both internal and external in response to challenges
- Understanding different regulation systems – Threat, Drive, Soothing, and when one may be more useful than another (Gilbert 2009)
- Taking a longer view over a period of time and using this awareness to consider what happens within the boom-and-bust cycle and during longer periods of symptom exacerbation (sometimes called a relapse or a setback)
- Making a bespoke plan of how to use a mindfulness-based approach in day-to-day life
- Developing awareness and attention to responding to specific difficulties with some therapist support (exploring this can be the basis of 1:1 sessions).

The course starts with noticing what happens when we bring awareness to the present moment; the food exercise and the body scan purposefully cultivate the 'paying attention in a particular way'. The role of intention is explored early in the group; the initial exercise on 'why am I here?', or what is more specifically asked, 'what are my hopes for the course and how could learning mindfulness help?', brings to light many reasons, such as: I want to be able to rest; My mind is very jumpy and I want more control; I want to be able to concentrate better; I want to be more compassionate to myself; I will do just about anything to get better so will give this a go.

The invitation at the start of the course is to be aware of the intention, hope (or longing) and then to let go and see what happens. This offers a number of things:

- It introduces the possibility of Being mode (chapter 8).
- The foundational attitudes of non-judging, patience, acceptance, non-striving, trust, letting go and beginner's mind are implicit.
- It undercuts discrepancy-based processing as the invitation is to be curious and potentially opens up the option that there is more to be experienced and learnt than we know right now.

Coming to the body

Mindfulness practices and inquiry start with the body as this is where the present moment is:

> The body thinks, but it doesn't think in words. Imagine being your own body for a minute? what would that be like? Up there is a head that thinks incessantly, eyes and ears are constantly monitoring the sights and sound with the outside world and a brain that is preoccupied so much of the time with responding to or planning how to act in or influenced the world… For the body, the basic units of information are not words or images but much simpler elements of experience which are most of the time beyond awareness. (Pole 2017, p.67)

In the practices, we are working with the body in a way the body can understand, we slow things down and experience through our senses. We are invited to drop beneath the labels, the names, the concepts and instead experience something simpler – the experience of the body: the different vibrations of the sounds, their direction, whether they are near or far, the volume, the pitch. In doing this, I become aware that although my ears hear the sounds, I can feel them resonate in my body: a softening in my right shoulder as the bird flies off into the distance. A gentle fluttering experience of sound behind my head and my back opens and drops down. A bracing sense when I hear some dogs barking, my breath quickens, then there's a pause and my breath deepens. I can also feel the silent space between the sounds, and this resonates with the pauses in my breath and a feeling of spaciousness in my belly.

Questions we can ask:

- What do I notice?
- What can I feel?
- What can I hear? – the tone, pitch, volume, direction. And where do I experience this hearing in my body?

- If I see something, going underneath the label and looking at its actual colours, shapes, textures – is a white wall all white?
- When we feel something, an emotion, we can ask: How do I know I feel that? Where do I feel that?
- What thoughts am I aware of? What do they make me feel? How do I want to act?
- Do I like or dislike this experience or am I indifferent?
- Is this familiar or unfamiliar?
- What do I make of this?
- What does it remind me of?

For example, if I say it's raining, I can then ask – how do I know that? And I might know that because I can hear raindrops pattering on the window, the temperature may have dropped and I can feel a change in the air pressure. I may also notice a lowering in my body and associate that with feeling fed up. And if I explore that, I find there is a heaviness in my lower body; I might see and feel a corresponding greyness in mood and particular thoughts associated with low mood and rain and greyness. I can then use mindfulness to explore this: the corresponding sensations in my body, a drop in my posture, sighing, a sinking feeling in my belly, and a heavy fatigue coming over my face and down my neck and shoulders.

And so what? What does this awareness offer us?

By recognizing how we feel, we can offer ourselves friendly compassion; for example, I can start to understand that actually when it rains my mood drops and it's not so much a mystery as to why this can happen. Then broadening out a little, I can start to experience my emotional states as a bit like the weather: when it's sunny and the sky is blue, I feel lighter, brighter, have a sense of opening and possibility. This also gives me insight into the reality that everything is in a constant state of change and flux: it won't rain for ever, I won't feel low for ever, I also won't feel bright and optimistic for ever, I'm always changing, like the weather. Gwyneth Lewis describes this shift from judging and evaluating to experiencing and describing:

> ...paying attention to the world around you, rather than wishing it to be different changes everything. Awareness allows the world to continue being itself without you raging at its refusal to conform to your will. It shows you the world as it moves, not in adjectives, but in verbs. (Lewis 2006)

Specifics of naming what is here

Going underneath concepts and labels immediately places us in an active experiencing and more precise place, reduces the tendency to be judgemental and offers opportunities for action. For example: 'I'm stiff and fatigued' can become – there is a feeling of stiffness in my lower back and a heaviness and lethargy in my legs, my eyes feel heavy… I find I can stretch and release the stiffness, support, close my eyes and actively rest for a while before going on to the next moment. In doing this, I can feel a sense of relief, a deeper breath and a lightening within my torso.

This specificity offers something important, an unhooking from the fixed sense of self to an awareness that *part* of me is stiff and heavy, another part of me can witness this and other parts of me are maybe experiencing sharp pain, a feeling of fullness in my belly; warmth in my hands. Labelling the experience in this way offers a few things:

- It enables us to turn towards; in other words, respond, not react.
- It allows us to see it is changing, and the sensations I have now are not going to be like this for ever.
- It opens up the experience – I can see this sensation is only part of what is going on now.
- It returns an element of control; part of me can see this – 'I can make some choices'; for example, choosing to rest, ask for help, put something off, or to sit or have a break rather than doing it how I've always done.

In other words, by noticing my body, feeling what is going on rather than labelling things and thinking about what I think about it or ignoring how I feel, or feeling overwhelmed by my mood, I can use my body to make small actions. In my example of feeling low when it rains, I can move in a different way, come out of a slumped posture and move around in a way that I know is invigorating and raises me up. Or I can soften and curl up and nurture myself, light a fire, make a cup of tea and read a book. Over time, I have noticed that recognizing this as 'rain' means my mood no longer drops as low.

Sharing with the group

In a group session, what happened in the practice is discussed and many find that through the sharing there is an understanding of that experience; but often something wider happens, there can be a glimpse into another way of experiencing and interpreting what is going on.

Hearing how others are responding and developing a more complex repertoire of possible responses within a trusted group environment of peers can change things. Again, Rhonda Knight highlights this in her account of Week 2:

> I was fascinated by the inquiry after the body scan, as people were mentioning themes that were similar to my doubts and struggles, and I realized that my

experience was not unusual. One particular fellow participant intrigued me, as they mentioned their awareness of pain during the scan, and how they could 'see' the shape and colour of the pain. This was beyond the realm of my previous thinking and experience as a nurse, who assessed pain from a medical model of practice, inquiring about the onset, characteristic and location of their pain. I never thought about assessing myself or viewing the pain that I experienced so visually. Listening to the other patients in the small group talking about their home practice was also helpful as I did not feel so alone in my daily commitment. Our sharing began the formation process of an incredibly supportive group that continued to meet independently for about 18 months after the programme finished.

BANANA MIND

'Banana mind' became a term used in the programme as the Zoom version required people to bring their own raisin for the 'food interaction exercise', AKA 'the raisin', and several people seemed to bring bananas! The raisin (or banana) is shorthand for mindful awareness: It can be a light-hearted exercise with a serious point as it fosters being curious; using the senses (including listening to food...); noticing thoughts as commentary on the situation and also memories; dropping (or noticing) being judgemental; being aware of bodily reactions, for example the automaticity of moving the hand to the mouth.

Inquiry to develop awareness

For us as clinicians, modelling curiosity and openness and using experiential inquiry rather than advice-giving or using a problem-solving or goal-focused approach sets a tone that that we are cultivating awareness and exploration to uncover what is already known somewhere. This may come up early in the group; for example, after the first body scan:

- Maria identified that while she started off feeling relaxed, as it went on she felt agitated and then exhausted.
- Wendy felt spaced out.

In the inquiry, we uncovered that Maria not only felt agitated, but she also responded in a particular way: she opened her eyes and moved and then went back to finding some comfort. She was also aware of trying very hard and that a 'giving up' followed the exhaustion. She reported feeling OK as she spoke and was curious about what happened but had doubts. We explored what she had done to look after herself and how that felt.

Wendy described her feeling spaced out as actually relaxing and pleasant, but this was unfamiliar to her as she would never let herself relax in the middle of a working day and didn't actually think she could. She reported feeling intrigued as to how she might use this.

These experiences led to a conversation about noticing what is helpful and supportive as well as noticing feelings and experience:

- In Maria's case, opening her eyes and moving, then making herself more comfortable by taking a deep breath and letting herself sink and let go of trying to 'do' the practice.
- In Wendy's case, exploring a sense of relaxation and considering the potential for more rest in her day.

In both these examples, the inquiry explored small actions and the use of the body to take care of the present moment.

Everything is an opportunity to learn and cultivate awareness, kindness and curiosity. These experiences can be explored, for instance curiously asking:

- What do you feel about that?
- What do you notice? About your reaction to this fact?
- Where do you feel this?
- What's it like? Is it familiar? What do you make of it?

The key is not to think about not doing the practices as being wrong, or even that it implies a lack of commitment. It is to be curious about the experience. How does this change things? There may be an activity pattern where it is hard to fit them in – what do you make of that? What do you notice about your pattern? How do you feel about that?

It may be that the practices have been forgotten, perhaps because automatic pilot is running things and they are not part of a well-established routine. What do you make of that? What is your emotional response to the situation? Is there guilt, frustration, sadness, resignation? What do they feel like?

Finding the time can be one thing, but many people report stopping and doing the practices is frustrating and difficult because they need to keep going, and stopping is actually painful. This is explored in more depth in chapter 15 on rest.

Noticing, naming and being with the reality of the situation can be a good first step and offers the opportunity to give ourselves compassion with the reality we are in and consider what we can do about it.

Inquiry into how and when someone is practising between sessions can illuminate challenges, as adding in mindfulness practices without making other changes can be difficult and sometimes uncomfortable. Learn to be gentle and learn from them. And come back to the body, what simple thing can change? It may be attitude – one doesn't need a tidy house to practise, it is possible to lie on the bed with eyes closed for 15 minutes rather than check social media…

Consider what this can offer:

- Posture – we spend so much time hunched over technology, this is placing the body in protective mode; finding a different posture of rest or alertness can change our moment instantly.
- Finding an anchor point – exploring where there is a sense of safety, perhaps it's the movement of the breath, maybe it's the rhythm of the breath, the movement of the belly or the back; or perhaps the warmth in the hands; the touch of the hands on the lap or cushion; the sensation of the bottom on the chair; the weight of the feet on the floor; or perhaps it's outside of the body, awareness of sounds outside, the sense of space and stillness in the room.
- Noticing tension and either dropping it where possible or accepting and taking care of it, moving as the body wishes.

This allows us to come 'offline', come away from thinking and enter the present moment. It creates a pause in the never-ending spiral of thoughts and allows us to rest and evaluate.

When it is time to resume activity, this can be done in a considered way having moved the body and established a helpful, perhaps less tense posture in which to carry on.

Specific challenges in inquiry into the present

Participants living with ME/CFS, fibromyalgia and Long Covid are presented with a challenge when facing symptoms of different levels of intensity – symptoms could be the day-to-day fatigue, pain, raised glands, nausea, sore throats and brain fog they currently live with, or they could be having a setback with more debilitating impact. The change in function can be quite extreme. To inquire into this skilfully it can be helpful to consider some cognitive processes experienced by all humans that may be affecting the reaction to a symptom exacerbation.

The human brain bases actions on a variety of data it continuously collects to keep us safe and functioning. When we come across a problem, the human mind is programmed to ask a series of questions:

- When have I met this before?
- What happened last time?
- What did I do?
- What is likely to happen this time?
- What should I do?

This is a subconscious and split-second questioning that is very helpful in many instances. However, it can become a problem when one has previously been debilitated for long periods of time and where 'recovery' means one is better than previously but certainly not *better*, and the symptoms keep recurring. The mind using this logic will identify a problem: 'I have these symptoms again; last time I had them I was really ill for three months, it took ages to recover; I had to go off sick for six months; I'm really worried that will happen again.' The individual thinking like this will most likely feel dreadful, and very likely stressed, and many people at this point find themselves doing *more* activity to prepare for the calamity that is ahead or push through and pretend it is not happening as they are so fed up with being ill.

A mindful inquiry in this situation offers several things:

- noticing the physical experiences as they are now
- noticing the memories
- noticing the feelings/emotions and thoughts
- noticing the *urge to act*.

This awareness may need to be built over time, but awareness can show what is going on right now and what is *not* going on now. There can be further questions based on an understanding of both the condition and the way the mind works:

- Is it likely I have the same infection?
- It's not, but do I have another infection? (And even if it is the same type of infection, it won't be the same experience because this is now, not then...)
- If I do have another infection, there will be signs and symptoms not usually present – high temperature, infected mucus, and so on. Then the option to take *action* arises: How do I need to take care of myself? The response to this question may be a new way of responding. Perhaps in the past there was a tendency to ignore all illness and crack on; maybe that's appropriate, but is it appropriate now? In this moment? What is needed *now*, to take care of myself?
- If not another infection, then what is likely? These fatiguing conditions ebb and flow; what is needed now to manage? To take care of myself?

In both cases, taking some time out resting might be an appropriate response, possibly rescheduling or reducing the energy requirements of a forthcoming commitment; for example, arranging to meet friends in a café at the end of the arranged walk or inviting a friend around instead of meeting out. Perhaps acknowledging what has been going on over the past few days/weeks – is there additional stress? Is sleep affected? Have I done more? How are my baselines?

Figure 11.2 shows how the concepts unfold and build upon each other through the course; in other words, the way we learn 'to pay attention in a particular way...in the service of self-understanding and *wisdom*' (Kabat-Zinn 2017).

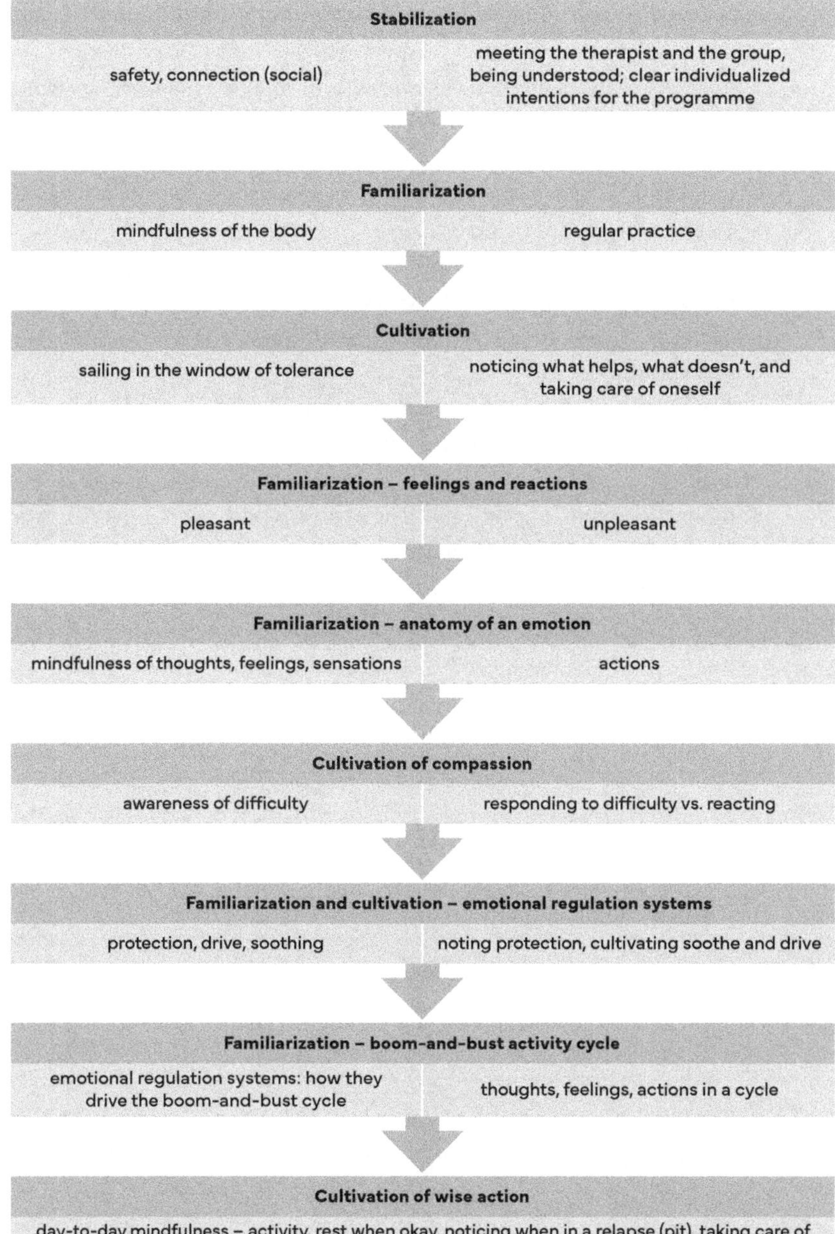

Figure 11.2 Familiarization and cultivation of awareness and wisdom throughout the course

SUMMARY

- 'Paying attention' is complex, requiring us to consider both the object of attention and the attitude to which we pay attention.
- Awareness in mindfulness involves cultivating an empathic curiosity about our internal and external experience.
- Inquiry into what happened and verbalizing what we noticed during an experience is a key part of the learning process.
- Doing this as part of a group can increase compassion for others and help us realize that we have common reactions and responses – our struggles and habits are part of being human.
- Teaching and learning in a mindfulness-based programme comes from the practice and inquiry, building on what is being said with additional information as required to reinforce understanding and the mindfulness-based approach.
- In managing long-term health conditions, noticing pain and fatigue as more specific sensations can be useful as this can allow subtleties and change.
- Enquiring into the specific experience can support people to take care of themselves gently and increase a sense of control.

Chapter 12

Mindful Movement

HOW DOES IT FEEL WHEN I MOVE?

With Sarah Nearney

- Challenges and benefits of incorporating physical activity
- Importance of this being a person centred and self-directed approach encouraging individual agency
- Guiding mindful movement and inquiry

Sarah Nearney has considered this from both a personal and professional perspective and shares her insights in this chapter.

Mindful movement is a component of all mindfulness courses, introduced as a formal practice in Weeks 3 and 4 but present throughout the course from the first practice where we engage with a small edible item. The hand moves, the eyes, the mouth and the head adjust as the focus of the practice changes. In the body scan, moving into a posture for a sustained practice, noticing where there is tensing, bracing, gripping and letting the body move to find ease. However, it is in the mindful movement practice that a longer formal session is dedicated to using movement and associated sensations as the focus of the mind's attention.

The practice cultivates this course's pivotal theme – namely *what is needed in this moment, and how I can invite my body to find its own way with kindness and compassion.* This session can result in rich and tender discussions around how bodies used to be, uncovering difficult emotions such as anger, frustration and sadness. Offering set or structured movements based on forms such as yoga, tai chi or chi gung can be challenging, perhaps because memories are evoked of how bodies may have once been or because they show starkly that even simple movements can cause pain or discomfort. For people whose bodies aren't doing what they used to do or what they want, this can be unfamiliar and counterintuitive.

Many come to us with histories of pushing their bodies, whether in job roles such as nursing where you keep going on long shifts, regardless of how you feel with no regard for breaks, or in sport where being able to push through pain and fatigue, working against those signals in pursuit of the goal, is part of the training. Those who do not have a history of systematically pushing through the body's signals to stop are now likely to find themselves restricted by fatigue and other symptoms in daily life, so that previously 'normal' daily activities are interrupted by intrusive symptoms. Janet described her fury at her body:

> 'I don't trust it, it lets me down, I need it to do what I want. When I have pain, feel sick and end up needing to go to bed I hate it, it feels like it's torturing me.'

Graded exercise therapy

Numerous participants in our programmes describe a complex relationship with exercise. While there is evidence suggesting movement or exercise can be very helpful in the management of patients with chronic pain or fatigue, it does need to be used skilfully. Many patients have followed the advice of health professionals, family and friends, as well as their own ideas based on prior experience, to push through symptoms and exercise regardless. This may have perpetuated a cycle of over-exertion and recovery, and in turn may have adversely affected other areas of life such as work or family. It may also have contributed to prolonged flare-ups and increased disability.

Finding a way through this can be delicate work for both the patient and their clinician, and may require different approaches in different stages. Recent qualitative research in the use of self-directed graded exercise came to several conclusions, including the need for bespoke guidance and therapies from health professional specialists in ME/CFS (Cheshire et al. 2020).

A participant who tried various ways of exercising and kept having to stop observed:

> 'So I'd do, you know, a hundred paces and then try and increase it. And I kept getting to, I don't know, like two hundred and fifty and then I'd stop, it would be too much. And because I was trying to go at my fifty paces at a time, so he challenged me and said, "Well what would it be like to just increase it by ten paces, or even five paces?"... And that was such a challenge for me... Because it can feel like, well if I can only do ten paces, extra paces, what's the point? But actually starting somewhere and just increasing by a little bit, eventually you will get, you know it's going to increase.'

Sarah's story

Sarah Nearney, a physiotherapist who first came to mindfulness as a participant and is now a mindfulness-based practitioner and teacher on the courses, describes her relationship to exercise:

'I had glandular fever when I was 42 and it knocked me for six. I had virtually a month in bed, or not moving very far from my bedroom if I got up. I didn't know much about fatigue, and about eight weeks after being diagnosed I decided that "enough was enough" and I'd better pull myself together. I still didn't feel great, but as I had never been ill for as long as this before I thought it was time to take action. On a cold February day in North Devon I decided that the best way was just to run this virus out of my body. I put on ankle weights (which I still don't know why I would do that now!) and started running. I ran four miles, which was the start of the beach to the end – it just felt like once I started I just didn't want to stop. However, when I reached the end I realized what a mistake this had been as I felt so ill. Having no mobile phone to call for help, I simply had to turn around and walk all the way back. It broke me, and I relapsed, being quite poorly for months afterwards.

'When I eventually managed to find some specialist help, I remember being asked what my hobbies were and struggling to think of any that weren't activity- or movement-based. I had been thinking of joining a running club. During the early days of pacing, and I suspect still at points now, I struggled to work out realistic goals for myself. When I asked about picking up my running again, I found it hard to think in small enough increments.

'It was suggested to me that I start with increments of one minute. I felt so frustrated with this – it didn't even feel worth getting changed into my running clothes! Slowly building up with a minute at a time was counterintuitive to me, I was used to diving in headfirst to things.

'Exploring using movements as part of my recovery has been so crucial to me. Perhaps more than any other practices on the course, mindful movement, which begins to be folded in from quite early on (from Week 3), has shown me my hidden patterns of thinking, reacting, responding.

'Using the notion of soft and hard edges, I have begun to consider how in other areas of my life I can work just around what feels that I am pushing or striving. I also see, by using the soft edges of movement, that my intention for activities is so important. For example, I tend to feel a personal sense of responsibility for things, people, tasks. It creates a strong pull towards me doing things that I can see need fixing. Using movement mindfully and exploring the edges of movement has also enabled me to find the even more tricky concept for me, which is what it feels to be in balance between the two edges.

'Recovering from the virus has taken years, but using activity that increased in increments, or layers, and exploring the notion of edges and the choice of where to work, has been so fundamental for me and with a very different focus to how I exercised before.'

NICE guidance

The latest UK guidance for ME/CFS (NICE 2021c) and Long Covid (2021a) has attempted to ensure that the individualized approach Sarah describes as helpful becomes more commonplace. This has meant removing graded exercise therapy based on a deconditioning model and delivered using fixed incremental increases in physical exercise from the guideline. Instead, it considers how individuals can incorporate sustainable levels of physical activity and exercise into their lives, bearing in mind what they wish to manage and having a flexible plan that may be very different to their previous approach to exercise. Establishing the physical baseline they are currently managing is an important part of the process and may require someone to look at how they 'exercise' in a different way. Other research reiterates the importance of patient autonomy, relevant physical activity and an approach that incorporates all elements of their life:

> Physical activity was experienced as helpful and enjoyable, especially related to leisure activities where flexible and individual adaptation was feasible. Non-customized activity may precipitate set-backs giving patients the impression of losing control and being betrayed by their bodies. Strategies to review energy usage in daily life could adjust expectations, diminish stress load and assist in approaching a more appropriate priority and balance. (Larun and Malterud 2011)

Long Covid and chronic pain (fibromyalgia) guidance reiterates the importance of adapting activity according to individual capacity and individualizing exercise advice accordingly (NICE 2021a, 2021b).

NIKKI

Nikki, a nurse practitioner who has had Long Covid for two years, started a slow phased return to work. After about ten months of slowly getting up to one third of her hours, she wanted to exercise more formally. In the first instance, it was helpful to get a measure of what she was doing on work and non-work days, so she kept a diary and measured her step count. Through this, she identified that she was doing more physical activity than she thought. This included a significant amount of steps on her work days; on her non-work days, she was managing housework, some gardening and online yoga three times a week. From tracking her activity, she then ascertained what she could manage regularly and started incorporating more walks into her days off and then added in more strengthening exercise into her yoga programme. Knowing her baseline meant that she knew what she could typically sustain, and if there were other things going on, she would reduce her extra 'exercise' and other activity if required. For example, she would sit down more at work, prepare simpler food that required less standing and ask her family to do more of the housework that week.

Being aware of physical activity and how one thinks about the activity is a key part of managing health conditions that include a post-exertional symptom exacerbation. The following participant observation describes someone reflecting on the role between setbacks and how they approach activity and exercise:

'I'm at a stage now where I can run, I can cycle. But sometimes I try and push it a bit much. And I end up going back. And I do get the physical symptoms again… So the thing really that causes the crashes now is just me thinking I can do more than I can. Physically.'

Mindfulness and the body

For most of us, there is a disconnect between ourselves and our body, seeing the two as separate. Somehow, 'I' am not my body: my body is something else, that in this case either does what I need it to do, or doesn't, and therefore needs to be corrected. Janet's quote at the beginning of this chapter that 'it lets me down, I need it to do what I want' is an example of this, where there is a conflict between the 'I' that wants to do something and the physical being. This is not an experience only associated with those who have health conditions, it is a common way to live. But if we think about it, it's extraordinary! We are our bodies: they are here every moment, our thoughts and emotions are expressions of our nervous and circulatory systems. We take in and encode images through our eyes and make sense of them using our brains. We talk of feeling heartened; we know what excited feels like; the agony of heartbreak and grief; the tense energy of fury. Finding a way to fully inhabit our physical beings is perhaps fundamental to managing not just a health condition, but all of our lives. Judging what can be done today, bearing in mind what I did yesterday and what I want to do tomorrow, as well as acknowledging what I may be dealing with – viruses, stress, poor sleep, etc. – is often unconsciously navigated. For the people who attend our programme, the physical reality differs hugely from how it used to be when they were in good health, and how they would like it to be. For many, the restrictions in daily life are severe. Being aware of this is challenging, and accepting it even more so.

Mindfulness invites us to notice what is happening, within our thoughts, our mood states and our bodies, so that we can embrace every aspect of our existence, both our physical and emotional selves. Deliberately turning towards and inhabiting the body opens up the possibility that we can reduce additional suffering. We can become more compassionate towards ourselves and in the process we may find something else, including pleasure, enjoyment and satisfaction.

The following comments from course participants capture elements of this:

'...it's made me more accepting of the fact that I do have chronic fatigue and this is something that, yeah, I can't just, if I just ignore it and try and plough on through that doesn't actually get me anywhere any faster! [laughs] And it's about kind of pacing and working with it, and although there is commitment, because of all that I do have a better quality of life. And yeah, just kind of letting go of some of those like expectations or kind of pressure that you put on yourself, um, to kind of work with it...kind of trying to find the like pleasure in being still and quiet for a while.'

'I *hate* my condition. I do hate my condition, but it's helped me to live with it more. And if I didn't have mindfulness then I would find it even more difficult to be able to, to live with it. Because the restrictions are, well. There are quite a lot of restrictions that put paid to social life and everything else, so. It is quite difficult from that point of view. But no, it's definitely helped me sort of mentally to cope with it all as well. And sort of physically, cause otherwise I think before I was always sort of constantly living on a knife edge with it and feeling so frustrated all the time.'

Mindful movement

All bodies move, even the breath itself is a movement. What makes movement mindful or different to everyday movements at work or home or during activities? The discussion at the beginning of the session in Week 3 can be emotive for participants and requires a different approach to movement than previously experienced. Memories may be evoked of past physical activities that have been enjoyable, satisfying or even an approach to dealing with stressful times in life: comparisons with a way of life they are currently not able to manage. The movement session may also bring up memories of attempts to recover, a desire to get better. Individuals may have attempted to take on board advice from health professionals, friends or family members who have suggested exercise as a way of recovering from fatigue but which did not lead to the promised outcome, perhaps because it was set at a too high level for their current state of health and led to setbacks. This may have also undermined confidence in any future form of movement, setting up future patterns of avoidance or resistance.

Movement becomes mindful when the individual can notice not only the sensation of the movement, which for some can be elusive or unavailable without some practice, but also the wider context of this movement. How do I feel about what I am feeling from the movement? Creating the conditions for participants to feel secure enough to notice this enables the wisdom to emerge, and the sense of agency to increase.

Mindful movement, with a gently inquiring and curious exploration of everyday movements, can reassure, provide space to reflect on what is lost and feared, and allow exploration of what is now possible. It is often a tender session where the awareness of the previous six weeks of practice is starting to show. Doing it in the second part of the session after two other practices, including anchoring where some movement or easing is encouraged and the discussion around noticing the sensations of pleasant events, seems to resource and feed this session too.

Which movements?

We offer a variety of movement approaches, each therapist working from their personal practice and clinical understanding. But the underlying ethos is the same: how we can use movement to draw alongside body sensations, whether they are pleasant, unpleasant or neutral; and how we can create the conditions for our participants to turn towards these with kindness and self-compassion.

One format is to use a structured approach based on the physiotherapy movements developed within the pain management programme that work through the whole body and exploring different ways to approach movement. For example, a person might explore turning their head by being curious about the experience of a very small turn.

The guidance is a blend between being both instructional and invitational. There is a cueing of the movement (e.g. an invitation to stand up), but this is balanced with exploration, personal agency and choice (what is it like to stand up now?). Each of the movements is considered sequentially; a pause and short rest is offered after the movement to notice and reflect. Choice points are offered of how to move in the next moment and perhaps consider alternative movements for the next moment rather than simply to repeat the movement in the same way. For example, to make movements smaller, bigger or smoother. There is always the choice of deciding not to move, or simply to let go and place a hand on areas of the body that are in pain or discomfort in a gesture of self-care and kindness. This can be a moment of great wisdom, and offering a profound insight into other areas of life.

Walking practice

Walking practices are common to many mindfulness-based programmes. In this course, walking practice is usually offered as part of home practice, especially if the course is online. A short walking practice of awareness walking that is already being done on a daily basis is encouraged. This involves bringing awareness to different parts of the body as it is moved, pausing and exploring being key teaching points. In addition, there can be invitation and investigation of other ways of walking, for example with strides that are longer, shorter, slower, asking where in the room we feel attracted to walk towards. Opportunities to stop and sit whenever that feels appropriate are openly offered, with a clear invitation to notice the urge to keep going with the group or to follow the 'instructions'.

Embedding inquiry into the practice

During the initial practices, inquiry is embedded within the movement practice and verbal feedback is encouraged, so the process unfolds with the participants being encouraged to be mindful of their thoughts as they move: 'What is it like to go part way? The whole way?' For example, opening and closing hands, what's it like to open as far as you can, but also what does the start of the movement feel like and the middle and where feels a good place for you to get to? Are my thoughts or feelings affected by my movements? How do I feel when I notice something I wasn't expecting? Or noticed before?

The movements of the neck and head, upper limbs and shoulders or trunk twists can be used as opportunities for finding starting and end points but also exploring the place in between. For many participants, this middle ground is very often rushed in an urge to get to the edge of stretch and sensation. The exploration of middle ground, in addition to some openness to discovering comfortable sensations associated with movement unique for each participant, interrupts the idea that we need to take things to their maximum in order for it to be worth something or to get benefit. The notion of what a satisfactory compromise may feel like within the body can thus be explored.

Often, participants reflect that they have never thought about movement or activity in general in this way, and the mindful movement practice can start to shed light on other areas of life where the person is operating within an 'all-or-nothing' mind-set. For patients with symptoms of fatigue or pain, this default mode can cause a vicious cycle that can then entrap, worsening the distressing symptoms.

Hidden patterns of thinking can show up vividly and be expressed in this session; for example, participants report making a fist so tightly that they marked their palms with their nails or stretched their fingers so much it hurts. Finding gentler, smaller or easier ways of moving is both interesting and satisfying, and offers a way in to movement that may be enjoyable and sustainable. The inquiry into how I am now, what feels a compassionate, friendly way to be with my body, echoes the previous sessions' work on anchoring: where do you find a point of stability now?

Exploring where there is a balance point or place to move into midline can be a rich area for growth if approached with kindness and self-compassion. Learning what it is to 'let go' may have only been glimpsed briefly so far by participants from focusing on their exhaling breath and its gentle, subtle letting go. With movement, we can start to see what it could be to respond to our body sensations, and what it is to take care of ourselves. I need to move more, I need to move less, I need to change position. This enables the group to explore choice points in a more embodied way:

- I choose to move more, I choose to move less, I choose to move in softer ways than I would have done.
- I allow myself a pause to check in, adjust or rest – moving more, moving less, the noticing of our first 'default' position, then an exploration of an alternative.

When working with fatigue, circumstances – events, people, life – can take over and we miss our own signs of fatigue or pain emerging. We feel embarrassed, we feel shame, we want to 'keep up' with others, we want to 'do our best' to 'do our part'. We resist, we fight against what is happening like a small child resisting bedtime, even though clearly tired. Patterns of thinking and behaviour that loop us, time and time again, back into patterns of thinking and feeling that lead us back into more fatigue or pain; into beliefs of personal responsibility that prevent us from stepping back and being overly optimistic about the number of commitments we can manage.

How can we create the conditions for movements to be mindful?

Mindful movement offers a way to practise making decisions to change the movement according to what is happening now rather than continue in well-practised grooves. Very often, participants notice discomfort, and their reaction is natural and understandable: they don't like it and they don't want it. They avoid by stopping moving, disengaging. They move because they feel that you have asked them to move, feeling that they are not in charge of their bodies, and do not have the power to say no. They are possibly not respectful of their bodies, and their bodies may not have been respected by others. As clinicians, we need to work with this power imbalance, being aware that participants may be keen to please us and hopeful that we can offer a solution. With mindful movement, we are offering a conversation not only between therapist and client but also between group participants, and most importantly with themselves.

Physical movements used in a mindful way teach us about 'hard edges': places of movement where strain or discomfort can be felt either in the place moving or indeed in other areas of the body that echo with the strain of moving – gritting teeth, stiff and tight neck muscles, for example. Or the 'soft edges', places where movements have just begun, places of intention perhaps or thoughts about what might feel right. It's a subtle place, and very often overlooked and unnoticed in the desire to move to the end of the range and the hard edge. This can uncover hidden patterns of thinking expressed in outward physical movements – ways of undertaking tasks or planning activities.

The following are questions that can be used to start the conversation about movement:

- What is our intention for our movement session today? How do we want to work? Is it softly, lightly, letting things wash over us today, or just being with others may be enough for today? Or is it with a little more curiosity, openness to movements that may have been more possible in the past and just haven't been recently?
- Within this movement I am doing right now, what range feels available to me? …to remain comfortable? …to be open to more expansive curious movement as if I was making this movement for the very first time?
- How does it feel to choose to stop and move into stillness?
- How can you make yourself 10% more comfortable, or even 5%?
- Can we reduce the effort the body is making? For example, do I need my jaw muscles to be tightly activated in order to sit on a chair? Does this allow me to find more alignment, poise or control in other areas of my body?
- Where can we allow ourselves to drop further into the support of the chair/bed/floor? Where can we allow ourselves to move into the space where we leave that support behind? For example, bringing our backs away from the chair, moving into space in front of us, noticing space that we create behind us, to the side, below or above us.
- How can we make movements more smoothly, and with greater ease?
- Asking with a kindly voice: Why is it we avoid these movements or the chance to use our bodies in this way? Is it frustration or shame, or a desire for them to be another way or as they were in a different part of our life?
- What are the thoughts we have as we move? Is it I wish I could move more? Or like I used to?
- What's the smallest movement you are able to make? What sensations can you feel?
- Noticing asymmetry: How do different sides of the body feel different?
- Noticing midline and moving away from midline and back again: How do we know that we are back in the middle?

- Pausing, breathing, resting. What feels the right thing to do after this?
- What is the quality of the movement? Has it got a steady feel? Is it jerky?
- How is the body now? Are you aware of judgements or comparison?
- What movements do you wish to make? What does your body need?
- Is this a familiar or unfamiliar movement or thing to do?

Movement practices using video conferencing

Using online video methods of communication such as Zoom does offer some challenges to teaching a movement-based practice, but there may also be some significant advantages. The challenges are probably more within the teacher/ therapist. It can be a very different way of working for a therapist who may be used to directing movement in certain predetermined ways in more usual, formal ways of teaching exercise. There may also be concerns about safety of movement. The tendency to want to 'do it right' can come up for the clinician, particularly if their background is in remedial physiotherapy or exercise, but this restriction can facilitate the invitational and self-management ethos of the programme as the participant is not in the room with an expert. Participants are invited if they wish to switch the camera off and to move within their familiar home environment. Emphasis is, of course, placed on moving safely, but the online nature and lack of the physical presence of the clinician helps to reinforce the fundamental theme of the practice, namely *the body contains the wisdom rather than the instructor*. It is up to the participants to move as they wish: they are autonomous.

The movement suggestions are offered simply as ways to notice different sensations that the movement brings and the response within the body or mind: 'I like this, I don't like this, this is boring, I want to do more movement, I want to do less', and so on. This can be a very uncertain place for patients who have been ignoring their own symptoms of pain or fatigue, or pushing through with long-held patterns of striving. The inquiry and conversational nature of the practice supports questioning and investigation and enables participants to verbalize their challenges, and their joys, through movement.

Link to activity

The movement practices are a link to how activity is pursued. Finding where we are now and inhabiting and exploring that place is a key element of the Being mode of mind (see chapter 8). It allows the brain to access more creative components; the fight/flight response with its reactive problem-solving solutions is calmed and more creative opportunities can sometimes arise. The following quotes are examples of how participants' awareness of the body and movement changed the way they engaged in activity throughout the day:

'I make a point [of taking] a photograph every day of one or other of the flowers, you know almost like a mindful moment… I look back on some of the little pleasure things that I'd recorded and one of those was light on ferns and I can still remember that feeling at the time and it's something I look for now, just the way that the light changes on ferns and stuff and it's…it's beautiful. And I can still do that. And that's, that can be almost like a whole-body experience.'

'…it made me aware of like this sort of competitive bit in you. And we were encouraged to notice that about ourselves, but then look. OK, so I don't have to push it that far to still get benefit from this exercise. And that's, that was a really good learning thing for me again I think. I mean I've had this for a while now, so I've got sort of slightly better at not pushing myself to crashing. But there are still times, you know, that you do.'

SUMMARY

- People with ME/CFS, fibromyalgia and Long Covid could have a complex relationship with movement and exercise. At the very least, the post-exertional nature of the symptoms means it can be difficult to judge how much movement is advisable.
- Clinicians need to be aware of the tendency of participants to follow instructions, perhaps to please the clinician or because they are familiar with a movement they have done before.
- There is a need to cue movements as guidance or invitations, rather than use directive or instructional language, and to use inquiry and investigation to encourage awareness of thinking processes that may be impeding optimal self-management (e.g. this is not worth it, it's so small, I need to do much more to get better).
- Mindful movement can be a powerful way to explore both habits in activity and new ways of approaching things.

Chapter 13

Mindfulness of Thoughts in Fluctuating Health Conditions

- The role of cognitive therapy in fatigue and pain
- Mindfulness-based approach to thoughts
- The role of thoughts in the boom-and-bust cycle of fatigue and pain
- Mindfulness-based group work and shared thoughts

Cognitive therapy in fatigue management

Cognitive therapies (such as cognitive behavioural therapy (CBT)) are an established way of helping people live with and manage their health from chronic pain to irritable bowel syndrome (IBS) and cardiac illnesses (Bernardy et al. 2018; Laird et al. 2017; Pizga et al. 2021), and this can include finding ways to manage thoughts and feelings. After all, anxious thoughts and feelings are unsurprising in people living with difficult symptoms that significantly impact upon their lives. Developing awareness of the role of thoughts and ways to manage them and their consequences is a part of living with a health condition that is not easily treated.

There has been some controversy over the role of cognitive-based therapies in ME/CFS, but after much debate the current UK NICE guideline defines it thus:

CBT for people with ME/CFS:

- aims to improve their quality of life, including functioning, and reduce the distress associated with having a chronic illness
- does not assume people have 'abnormal' illness beliefs and behaviours as an underlying cause of their ME/CFS, but recognizes that thoughts, feelings, behaviours and physiology interact with each other. (NICE 2021c, para.1.12.32)

Mindful awareness, and the cultivation of supportive helpful ways of being, supports people in identifying the interaction of thoughts with behaviour and physiology. A mindfulness-based approach will use practices to calm and soothe the system, which can ease symptoms of anxiety as well as pain and fatigue, but also enables the emotional brain (whose main function is protective) to 'calm down'. This then enables different perspectives to arise that may help constructive adaptation to the situation.

The rest of this chapter explores the nature of the thoughts that can be identified in fluctuating fatiguing conditions and how this awareness can support compassionate and constructive ways of living with and managing the condition.

Mindfulness-based approach

The mindfulness approach to thoughts is perhaps different to what we normally use. It is not about positive thinking, changing thoughts or even doing anything with them at all. It is more about treating thoughts as events, perhaps in much the same way as we experience sounds. For example, if we hear sounds we are aware that some sounds we like and some sounds we dislike, we know that sounds come and go and that we can experience relief, for example when drilling stops. Could thoughts be treated in the same way? We experience many thoughts every day; some of them are not even our own, they can come from what others have said today or in the past, what we may have read or seen in the media, and so forth.

With mindfulness of thoughts, instead of paying attention to the content of our thoughts, we watch the thoughts come and go perhaps like clouds across a blue sky or as if we are standing behind a waterfall and watching the water torrent in front of us. Some people find it useful to imagine they are watching their thoughts as if they were on a screen in the cinema; this metaphor is helpful as terrible things can happen on a screen but the screen itself is not damaged; we turn off the television or change channels and different images are there.

Thoughts in more detail

Thoughts are phrases, images and other mental events that come and go, albeit some are more charged emotionally, some compel us to action, and others are mundane or at times tedious and often repetitive. One of the first things that stands out when people learn a mindfulness practice is that thoughts are noisy, jumpy, intrusive and seemingly random. A lot of energy can be expended in a struggle with them, and anxiety can arise when the thoughts either won't do what we think they should (in many cases we think thoughts should go away while the breath is attended to) or tell us things that sound like facts.

Thoughts, however, are complex and have a subjective context, and one of the things humans always do is add a layer or interpretation to it that creates an emotional charge. For example, a night out is being arranged and at the last minute a text arrives from Gabi, one of the party, saying 'I can't come, sorry'; the other three people have different reactions:

- Jane feels concern and thinks 'Oh, I hope she is OK' and texts her back asking for more information.
- Mini feels neutral and thinks 'Never mind' and texts 'I'll see you next week'.
- Lucia feels irritated and thinks 'She's done this before, she's unreliable' and does not text back.

Their reactions are unique and based on multiple variables: including how they are feeling at the time based on their personal history of relationships generally, what is going on in their lives and what has happened just before the text, as well as on their individual and particular relationships with Gabi.

Awareness of thought and the mind

Mindfulness-based courses start by establishing a stance of seeing thoughts as events that come and go. Seeing that thoughts are just thoughts and that there can be numerous ways to respond is a useful way to start to change the relationship to thoughts. We can feel freer and not so bossed around or overwhelmed by them. This is developed by creating 'a place' from which to observe that encourages the sense that 'we are not our thoughts'.

The existence of thoughts and the quality of mind in which they arise is apparent as soon as someone starts to practise. Attention is placed in something tangible, for example the breath or footfall when walking, and the practice is to be aware of the object of attention but also the nature of this jumpy, seemingly random mind.

Mindful awareness allows us to see that:

- thoughts, to some extent, have a life of their own
- the present moment consists of far more than thoughts and is quite likely *not* what we think it is.

We can touch into *how* we are: perhaps preoccupied; finding it hard to settle; feeling perturbed by something; or feeling calm and relaxed and sleepy. While some states might be preferred, there can be an opportunity for choice arising from this awareness:

- If the moment is perceived as pleasant, to appreciate it, take it in (Hanson et al. 2021).
- If unpleasant to:

1. be aware it can change
2. identify ways of compassionately caring for oneself, which can include how one thinks.

This experience of touching into sensation, seeing thoughts as passing events and the lived current experience, can be both soothing and empowering.

MBCT focuses on the relationship we have with thoughts and the feeling that 'gives birth to the thought' (Segal et al. 2013, p.307) and explores that relationship rather than trying to adapt the content of the thoughts.

For example, in the third group session, Amina declared: 'I'm really fed up, this is really difficult, my thoughts are really getting in the way of my enjoyment and rest. This isn't working.' We explored how she felt, physically and emotionally, offering an opportunity to accept her thoughts, be curious about them and bring awareness to the whole of her experience. She identified feeling physically and mentally fatigued, which were aching limbs, sore throat and headaches, and difficulties concentrating. She was irritated and frustrated, which felt scratchy, and she was aware of abdominal tension and a tightness in her face and shoulders. After some time being curious about all of this together, others in the group joined in recognizing this feeling and thought as a familiar state to many of them. Amina reflected at the end that her relationship to the experience of the intrusive thoughts changed in several ways:

- She felt pleased that she had been able to express how she felt honestly and that the group and the facilitators had appreciated how she felt, that she was not 'doing it wrong' and that the practice was not 'failing'; in fact, she now felt that noticing *how* she felt *was* the practice.
- Doing this was both interesting and fruitful, as during the discussion she observed a bigger process and identified that she had had a busy week, was out of her usual routine in the summer holidays and had not slept well.
- During the conversation, she identified that she was irritated that the symptoms were there and that she had other, more challenging thoughts and feelings underneath: 'My Long Covid symptoms were getting worse' and 'I am never going to get well'.

The thoughts that she couldn't do this and it wasn't working were thoughts that arose from how she was feeling, and while at first difficult and very uncomfortable, observing them and being aware of the feelings gave rise to a potentially more compassionate stance. She was able to look at the thought 'I'm never going to get well' and immediately identify that she had come a long way – from being in bed for six months to now going out most days – and identify that she'd had an increase in symptoms because she was doing more and it was understandable that she was irritated and fed up, and perhaps she needed to slow up for a few days.

Amina's thoughts were actually part of her symptoms; by noticing them and the feelings, and what may lie beneath the thoughts, she was able to feel better and also choose to act in different ways. Learning to see thoughts for what they are, unhooking from them, can be a significant part in managing a health condition.

Once we are able to relate to thoughts as events, we can, like Amina, start to look at their content and what they may mean. While this is individual, it can be useful to realize that a lot of our thoughts are not personal, and many others have very similar thoughts arising from similar health conditions, to the extent it may be useful in some cases to see the thoughts as another symptom of the health condition.

Sharing common thoughts

Managing how we think and feel is increasingly part of how healthcare is delivered. There are studies that have looked at the specific thought processes and cognitions with people who have a particular condition, such as diabetes, IBS, cancer and cardiac illness. Some work has been done on the specific thoughts of people with ME/CFS (Surawy et al. 1995), and a list was generated for use in mindfulness-based groups. We have added to it over time based on clinical experience and the feedback in the groups. Sharing that these thoughts are common can be very moving, and I have been accused (jokingly) of being a mind reader. Interestingly, this has become more powerful in online delivery as it is shared as a slide we work on together. Seeing the thoughts as part of the condition and seeing immediately that others think like this has been pivotal for many people in their relationship with their illness. Experiencing it as part of the group experience, we hypothesize it can undermine the struggle of many people's shame and guilt about their condition and their thoughts about themselves.

Common thoughts reported by people with fatigue and pain conditions (adapted from Surawy et al. 2005):

1. I'm tired and achy now, so I'll feel like this for the rest of the day.
2. Other people's needs are more important than mine.
3. There's no point starting this unless I can finish it.
4. I should always do things really well.
5. Everyone else would do this activity better than I am doing it.
6. I'm not the person I was.
7. It's better not to talk to anyone about how I am feeling, it might upset them.

8. I should be able to cope with this.
9. I can't do this as well as I used to.
10. How am I going to get everything done? I've got so much to do.
11. I feel tired, but it would bother me if I left the job half-done, so I'll finish it anyway/not start at all.
12. I must be careful what I do today, in case I feel worse tomorrow.
13. Taking breaks is a waste of time, I should be able to just keep going.
14. I feel better today, I need to catch up.
15. I feel better today, there's nothing wrong, I'm just lazy.
16. I feel unwell, I'm back to square 1.

From the above list, it is possible to identify where in the boom and bust they fall. A group activity we do is to work through the thoughts, and consequences of the thoughts, and populate a slide (or whiteboard) with thoughts and consequences (see Figure 13.1). From generating this on a slide/whiteboard, the group then moves to talk about what could be the choice points once we have observed the cycle and the associated thoughts and consequences. How can we bring mindfulness to these moments and what does awareness offer at these times? (See Figure 13.2.)

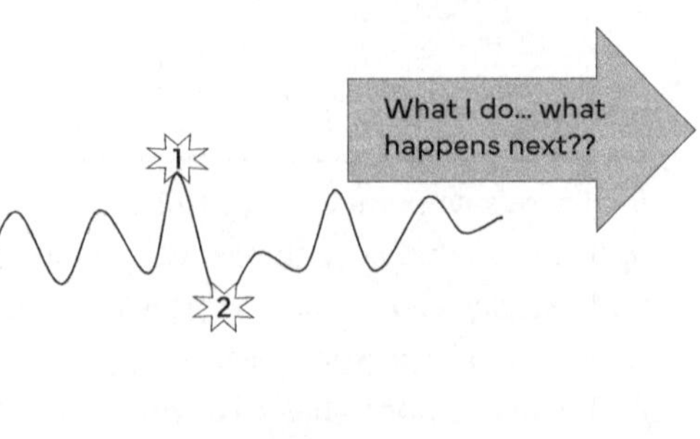

Figure 13.1 Thoughts in the boom-and-bust cycle of fluctuating health conditions

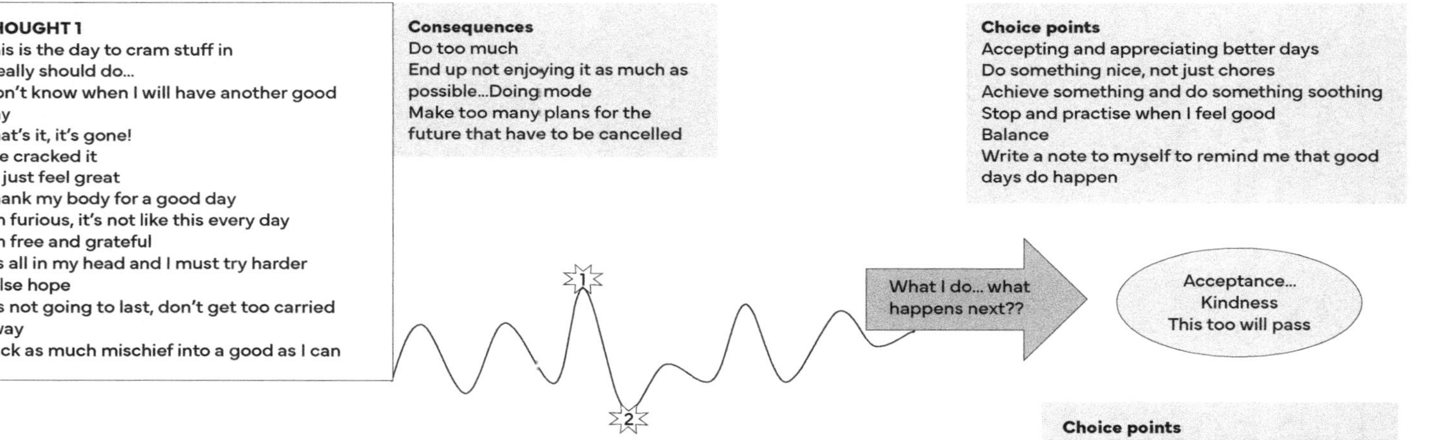

Figure 13.2 Consequences of the thoughts in the boom-and-bust cycle

These ideas may have been explored in other ways earlier in the service, so the observation of the thoughts and consequences and the choices available are looked at through the prism of mindful awareness, that is to say, awareness with a particular quality of flavour including non-judgement, patience, compassion and kindness, as well as trust that there is often another way. This goes back to the initial definition of mindfulness and the mechanisms described by Shapiro et al. (2006): attention, attitude and intention that allow a 'reperceiving' of the situation and different choices to emerge. From this, it is possible to develop new ways of thinking that are supportive and kind and allow the situation to be navigated with awareness, understanding and choice.

Thoughts and the emotional systems

In previous sessions, the three emotional regulation systems (see chapter 8) will have been referred to. Some participants find it can be helpful to look at how their thoughts can be driven by different systems, how there can be a particular texture to the thinking. Tables 13.1 and 13.2 simply classify some of this. Notice how Drive can lead to either Soothing or Threat. Drive can be the way that a more compassionate approach can be activated; for example, scheduling rest, planning achievable goals and being able to spot both thoughts, feelings and behaviours and what may be underneath them. This awareness can lead to more choices and options despite the challenge of the boom-and-bust cycle.

Table 13.1 The emotional regulation systems in the 'boom' of activity cycling

BOOM	Thoughts	Feelings	Actions
Threat	I've got to get this all done now because I won't have much time. I've been so lazy. What will people think of me?	Shame; guilt; disgust; fear. Feel tense and stressed; tightness in the body; pain.	Keep going despite feelings; suppress. OR Give up in despair; shut self off, don't accept help.
Drive	I want to get this done; I feel more like me; this is satisfying; I need this to be as good as or better than (other person).	Buzz; excitement; enjoyment; sense of achievement.	Keep going until I can no longer manage; plan more activity – e.g. events in the future (may tip over into Threat once I cannot keep up).
overdrive	I'll miss out if I don't... Next I will...	Speed; agitation; can't sleep; wired.	
Soothing	I'm enjoying feeling well and the fact that I can do this. I'll make sure I do it in the best way for me.	Pleased; content; calm.	Either stop at a point it's helpful to stop, or if I can't or don't remember to, then will plan a break and rest. Ask for help.

Table 13.2 The emotional regulation systems in the 'bust' of activity cycling

BUST	Thoughts	Feelings	Actions
Threat	I feel so alone; this is awful, it's just like last time (memory of being very ill); I'll never be well.	Tension; tightness; fear; anger.	Hide away; shut others out. Tip into Drive to 'fix' the problem.
Drive	I must take control and put my plan into action/ find the answer. Problem-solve.	Determined; resolute; motivated.	Organize, set goals – OK if appropriate. Look for cures, go on internet.
overdrive	There must be something someone can do. Ruminate.	Wired; agitation.	Tip into Threat when no result.
Soothing	This is familiar. What can I do to take care of myself? This is hard, be gentle. Notice when mind goes to the past – keep thoughts present. Notice what may have led to increased symptoms.	Use mindfulness and be open to all feelings – good or bad; allow bad feelings – symptoms, tension – to be there. Notice what's OK; recall others who feel like this.	Rest; gentle movement; ask for and accept help; mindfulness and compassion practices. Work on a lower baseline. Notice when improvement starts.

Mindful awareness is not necessarily about being in the Soothing system, it is about being able to see which system one is in and the components of this moment that may be helpful or unhelpful; and making some change, whether it is doing something differently or thinking about it differently. Or perhaps the wisest thing can be to let it be and see what arises. Acceptance of how things are and what this opens up is commented on by a participant:

> '…just being more accepting. Instead of thinking, um, you know constantly aware of all the stuff I can't do, being more aware of what I can do. Cause you can mindfully be aware of where my mind is going and make a choice; am I going to concentrate on the fact that like there's loads of stuff in the garden that I can't do? Or am I going to concentrate on the fact that there are flowers in the garden and I can actually appreciate them. I can look at them and I can still take them in. You know. So, things like that in terms of like the fatigue and stuff, and not, I don't know what the right word is. [long pause] Not striving in maybe the same way? So, being more accepting of, just what is.'

Learning about oneself and the thoughts and feelings that are normally private and usually go unnoticed can be shared in a group setting, and are perhaps best summed up by a participant:

'But actually going to the classes and being involved in a group allowed me to see what others were going through. And I was able to compare myself. To a certain degree. But then also not to feel guilty. Or feel that I shouldn't be there. So it was good for me to be kind to myself... And historically I was never very good at opening up. And this really, really helped me to open up. And talk about things that normally just go on in here [indicates towards his head in circular motions], or have gone on in there for many years, so. Yeah, I think, that was probably one of the biggest things that I've learnt.'

SUMMARY

- Many thoughts that people with fatiguing and pain conditions have are similar and can be part of the boom-and-bust fluctuating nature of the condition.
- A mindfulness-based approach allows people to see their thoughts, and also the feelings and symptoms that may give rise to the thoughts, and then respond to them in a chosen way (rather than habitual or automatic reactions).
- A group approach (or understanding others with a similar health problem think the same way) can be supportive and potentially reduce self-blame and guilt and increase a sense of self-management and coping with the health conditions.

PART 3

Applying a Mindfulness-Based Approach to Life

Mindfulness can be used to inform daily life. As an occupational therapist, I have used this approach to inform the self-management approach used in ME/CFS, pain management and Long Covid.

Mindfulness is often regarded as 'the meditation practice'; however, while the meditation practice enables practitioners to observe themselves and to practise skills such as attending with curiosity and compassion, mindfulness offers a whole approach to life and a way of dealing with and living with challenge. Living with a fluctuating health condition and its consequences is not easy, and to be of most benefit, we need to consider how mindful activity can support the adaptations people often need to make. This approach is more than 'mindful moments' or mindfulness of an activity, it can be a fundamental shift in how one approaches life, and it seems that this is most efficacious when combined with formal practice (Crane et al. 2014; Ribeiro, Atchley and Oken 2018).

Part 4 considers activity management and how mindfulness-based processes can support activity management. Then how mindfulness can support rest, including the challenge people have with resting.

Chapter 14

Mindfulness-Based Activity Management

- Day-to-day mindfulness
- Activity cycle – boom and bust
- Energy requirements of activity
- Feeling tone and energy management
- Underlying regulation systems and the impact on activity and energy.
- Managing setbacks
- Wider participation
- Applying the approach – a case example

Day-to-day mindfulness

Mindfulness-based stress reduction and mindfulness-based cognitive therapy courses (Santorelli et al. 2017; Segal et al. 2013) all include mindful activity; in fact, the first practice is an activity, mindful eating. By using a daily activity and the connection with the object and the activity, the approach is immediately applicable to other things we do throughout the day. The idea is that everyone tries out something every day, be it brushing teeth, a few sips of a cup of tea, a key in the lock, walking around the house, or whatever they wish. Mindfulness of daily activity can immediately start to change the relationship one has with activity, and a more embodied presence, doing one thing at a time, even if only for a few minutes, can feel soothing and enjoyable as well as show up patterns of reaction. When I did my first mindfulness course, I realized I gritted my teeth every time I got out of bed. Becoming curious about this and exploring my movements and bodily tension has changed this additional tension in my life.

Mechanisms of mindfulness in action

Shapiro's three axioms of mindfulness, Intention, Attitude and Attention (Shapiro et al. 2006), introduced in chapter 5, can be helpful when we consider what we are doing in daily life as much as in a practice.

For example, I am typing this, aware that I am a bit tired after a full day at work in clinics. I'm digesting my dinner (aware I probably ate too much); and my daughter is texting me. But I want to place *attention on the words* I am writing, and in order to do so I take a deep breath and focus on my computer and my body. I can feel the laptop on my legs and feel, see and hear the keys as I type. My awareness wanders off to my daughter, my digestion and my tired back. *My intention* is to finish this paragraph. I absorb myself in typing my thoughts, adjust my body and set a length of time to write. *My attitude* consists of a determination to write this, and at the same time doing it with compassion for my tired body (and grumbling stomach), so I won't do it for too long. I am also aware of my daughter's needs. This is moment-by-moment awareness of the activity, and by being absorbed in it I can find it less fatiguing. But by being aware of the other demands, I can place my awareness intentionally in different places.

This process is built into practices like the body scan, where we purposely move attention around the body, drop attention from one area and then move it to another.

Attention is also developed as a broader sweeping awareness – in my example I am aware of all the things that potentially could take my attention; I sweep through my experience, then choose to focus on one area. I can take care of myself by periodically checking in with the other areas, then directing my attention in a more single-minded way.

This awareness can lead me to manage the present moment and enables me to switch from one moment to the other. It could also enable me to identify what is underneath some of this: Why am I working at this time? What was it that led me to eat too much? And overall, how am I planning my time?

These could be helpful questions, or they could be an example of overthinking. As a one-off event, it's OK, I'm busy and rushed things today, and I know that I have a busy mind that throws up thoughts I want to capture for this project. However, if self-care and parenting keep coming in second or third place after work, what does this mean? And is it how I want to live?

This broad awareness is perhaps not the same as doing several things at once nor is it multi-tasking: it is *switching attention in a conscious intentional* way from one activity or experience to another and *making choices*. This is intentional action, rather than being driven to compulsively do one thing or feeling that other experiences are demands that need to go away or be dealt with before I can get to the writing. Of course, at times I will need to set aside longer periods of time to write, when I clear time and communicate the need to work to others. I may do other things that support this like turning off wi-fi and my phone and making sure I have appropriate seating (and not eat too much!).

Formal practices informing daily life

The above sounds very much like my meditation practice; I may do short anchoring and checking-in practices and longer, more sustained periods of meditation, including going on retreat. The longer periods of practice/writing mean I can do the shorter ones, and the shorter ones also keep me going and show where I am and perhaps what needs some work.

The 'formal' practices can also start to enhance daily life; for example, body scans can help sleep and rest and also support creating space to rest in the home environment as practising at home is a requirement of the course. Interestingly, the switch to online courses during the pandemic enhanced this as it required people to be on their own in a room, preferably with the ability to lie down comfortably while attending the course. However, we are aware it may well also be a barrier to practice and attendance. Short pauses, although taught as a routine practice initially, start very early on to be used to ground in situations of duress.

Daily life informing formal practice

Early application within day-to-day life has several benefits to the course. There is an immediate application of skills that are relevant and of help instantly, both to the individual and to the collective process of learning within a group. The benefits in daily life mean there is more motivation to continue with the longer practices that fuel this new way of being and the emerging skills. The group environment with space to talk about the home experience reinforces this as people share what they are noticing and trying. The practice used in this way can create the potential for a positive cycle of applied learning to occur as people try things out and find it useful; then the formal practice becomes more alive and relevant (see Figure 14.1).

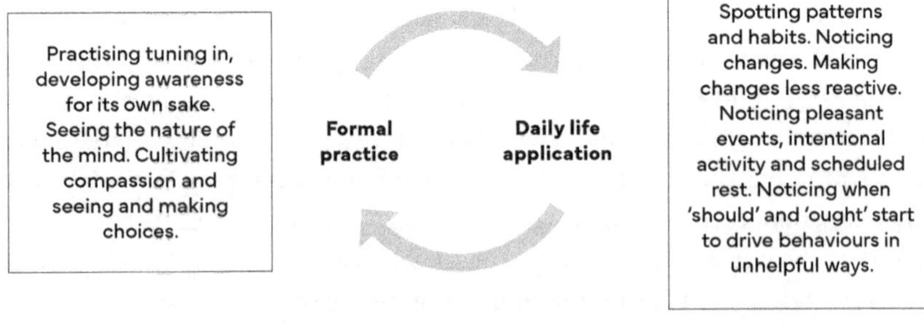

Figure 14.1 How daily life application and formal practice work together

Activity management is a strategy used by many people living with health conditions; arguably everyone uses it, but having a health condition means it may not be possible to do everything, and previous patterns of activity and methods of doing something may no longer be practical. There is also significantly less scope for 'winging it' or pushing through, as the recovery period can be intrusively long and painful and disruptive to other areas of life.

People often report that they have days when they can do a little more, but that is when they can find themselves on a treadmill of exertion followed by recovery. While mindfulness is not a cure, many people find that the mindfulness-based approach helps them gain control, take care of themselves more effectively and feel better about their situation.

People with fatigue often describe having varying amounts of symptoms from one day to another or even within the same day. This can make it difficult to decide whether to attempt an activity. Most people (understandably) tend to do more when they feel a bit better and not as much when they feel unwell. They can find that this means they 'overdo it' one day and then have several days recovering. This can lead to big swings in activity over time – the 'boom-and-bust' approach or 'activity cycling' (described in chapter 3).

Problem with listening to the body

The signals that the body produces in long-term fatigue are not the best guide to what we should or should not be doing 'in the moment'. This is very different with acute as opposed to chronic conditions, such as having a stomach bug. With an acute infection, the body reacts by making us feel unwell so that we rest more. When we feel better, this is a sign that the illness has passed and we can get going again. Longer-term fatigue is different from an acute illness: listening to the body on a moment-by-moment basis to decide what we should or shouldn't do is often unreliable. The body can feel deregulated with sleep and eating patterns as well as activity levels being highly variable. A longer view of what I am doing now, what I have done and what I will need to do bearing in mind what I understand I can do is required and is complicated. Time, patience, compassion and possibly some help are required to find a way through this.

Activity analysis

Finding a way to gain control of this challenging situation takes time and some thought. The phrase 'activity management' is used as opposed to 'energy management' as the focus is on the activity and how that can be managed. This is because we can manage our activity, and while we hope energy may improve this way, we cannot guarantee it will. However, achieving activity-based goals can increase the sense of having more control and enables participation, improving well-being.

Being able to analyse what we do and what may be impacting on our energy can of itself change things, and then it is possible to respond with considered use of scheduling or, when this is not possible (because some things just have to happen), of adaptations that may be useful. Mindfulness offers a way to notice and reflect and choose ways of responding to the observations. It can also help with the emotional component of the process; how we feel about an activity is subjective and based on personal preference and history.

Here we will look at:

- Activity levels (high, medium, low and rest)
- Patterns of activity (over a day/week/month, boom and bust)
- Tone of activity (like/dislike/neutral/mastery)
- Texture of activity (underlying flavour or 'texture' – Threat, Drive, Soothing).

Activity levels: Ascertaining the demand of an activity

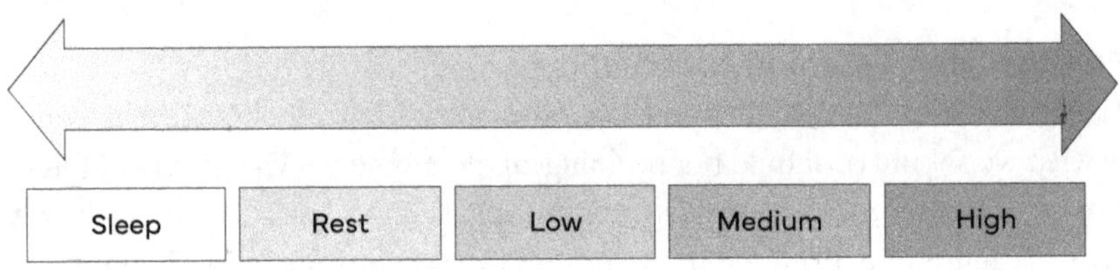

Figure 14.2 Continuum of activity levels (adapted from Cox 2000)

Activity levels are on a continuum (Figure 14.2), and while sleep is included here, it is for the purpose of looking at the pattern of activity, as we know that many people with fatigue find it unrefreshing as well as problematic. Rest is complex and has its own chapter (chapter 15). How one works out what is high, medium or low is another matter. The principle is that the demand is the same on either a good day or a bad day, except that on a good day it will feel easy and the temptation to do loads of high-level activity will be strong. On a bad day, something high may well feel impossible. One way of thinking about this is to compare it to calorie counting – a confectionery bar always has however many hundreds of calories whether we have eaten two and a roast dinner or just had salad. So if a shower is a high-level activity, it is recorded as that *regardless* of how we feel at the time. This is quite tricky (and I suggest any clinician suggesting activity diaries to anyone has a go at it…). However, many people we see do manage this, and Figure 14.3 is an example diary that shows a boom-and-bust pattern of activity as well as a deregulated sleep pattern.

How can a 'boom and bust' approach to activity be changed? An awareness of abilities and limitations can enable people to plan the way that they use their energy through prioritizing things they must do and would prefer to do. This can take a period of reflection, testing and problem-solving before a solution can arise, as exemplified by Sindra and Carlos.

SINDRA

Sindra is a single parent who worked full-time and liked gardening and running. Since contracting Covid she has reduced her work to part-time from home and had to go on Universal Credit. She has had to stop running completely and has friends and neighbours help with bigger gardening tasks, such as cutting back shrubs and mowing the lawn.

She prioritizes looking after her home and children and maintaining her job, albeit on reduced hours.

She got to this after a process of trial and error; on a better day she mowed the lawn and realized this meant she was not able to clean the bathroom or go to work and struggled with the school run for a couple of days. She became very aware of the need to prioritize and work not just within her capacity for the day but also bearing in mind other tasks and responsibilities going forward.

She also realized that while the garden was important, there were other elements she could do. She entered into an agreement with a neighbour who was very happy to help with mowing in exchange for the seedlings Sindra grew and help with their weeding at times as they found kneeling difficult.

CARLOS

Carlos really enjoyed hosting dinner parties, but after contracting glandular fever and developing ME/CFS and being off work for 18 months, he was not able to both cook and host in the way he liked. Other areas of life were becoming more manageable, and he had started back at work on a reduced hours contract. But after trying to cook in the way he enjoyed, he found he would have to cancel the event at the time as he felt so unwell or be in bed for days and be off work sick afterwards.

After a period of reflection he realized that what he really enjoyed was getting friends together, even if he was not able to cook for them. He started inviting small groups of friends around for cheese and pudding parties, which were a lot of fun but much less work to prepare. He also found it worked best if he set time limits, so he made everyone aware that the evening would finish by 10pm and that they could help by bringing food and drink and help him clear up before they left.

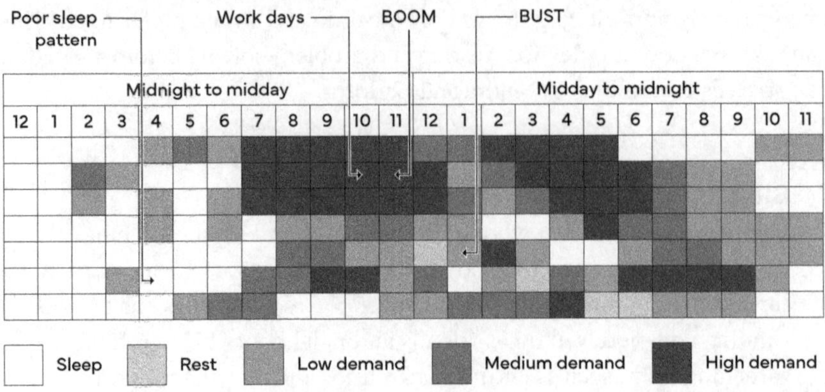

Figure 14.3 Liz's activity diary

These solutions that Sindra and Carlos worked out do not happen easily and require a significant degree of acceptance and self-knowledge as well as resource and communication with others, all of which can be challenging when one is not feeling well.

Mindfulness and observation

Observation in mindfulness has certain qualities that can support how the diary sheets are approached: non-judgemental awareness; curiosity; openness; trust. In other words, some of the attitudinal foundations of mindfulness (see chapter 5).

Noticing in this way is potentially taking a compassionate stance. There is an increasing awareness of the cycle of fluctuating activity levels and corresponding reactions and responses: perhaps a sense of enjoyment and urgency when on the upturn followed by disappointment, fear and anger when symptoms return and there is a prolonged and uncertain time of reduced capacity. After a while, people can start to see what may be driving the cycle and perhaps consider this.

The inquiry used throughout the practices on the mindfulness course is 'What do I need now?'; asking this at the end of a practice encourages wisdom and compassion and when applied in daily life can perhaps be a way of noticing drivers such as guilt and loss, or simply habitual ways of going about life, as well as a sense of uncertainty as to how to address the situation. We see people move from awareness at each stage, which can be very uncomfortable as patterns are recognized. Ingrained habits and pressure on time can create little energy or space to see what changes could help. This reduced capacity can hold people in repeating patterns.

Mindfulness can reveal this process through pausing to reflect and consider choices. We may then see the boom-and-bust cycle slow up, or at least be consciously managed. For example, choosing to do a higher-level activity but preparing beforehand and making time for recuperation afterwards.

Setbacks can come due to illness, stress or exertion, or sometimes just happen.

The post-viral state in some means there can be fluctuations when the body produces symptoms for no particular reason. Sometimes, it is wise to investigate why there may be a setback; other times, accepting it is part of the condition and needs to be managed is the best thing. There is more on setbacks later.

Over time and with practice, the sense of wisdom and awareness can take more of a central role and there can be a feeling of control as the boom-and-bust cycle is observed and self-care, planning, resting and pacing strategies are implemented (Figures 14.4 and 14.5). After some work, an activity diary can represent this change; in Figure 14.6, sleep is not perfect, but there are clear breaks, rests and high-level activity is spread throughout the week.

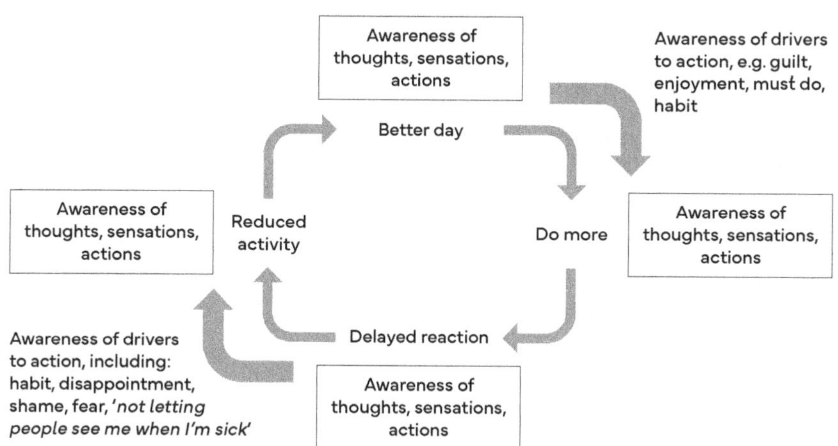

Figure 14.4 Mindful awareness of the activity cycle

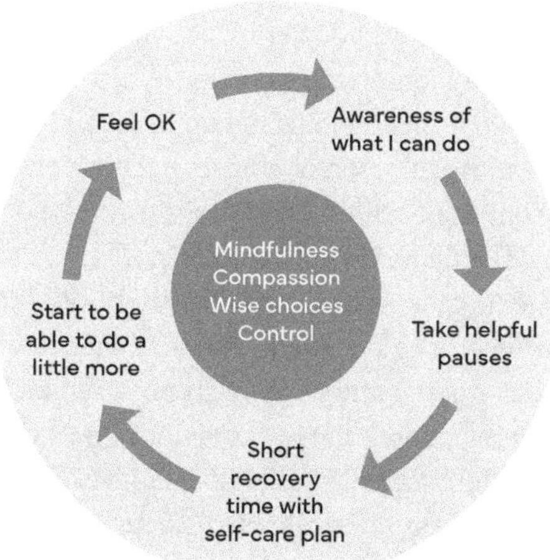

Figure 14.5 Boom and bust: calmed so there is less need for recovery time and an ability to do more

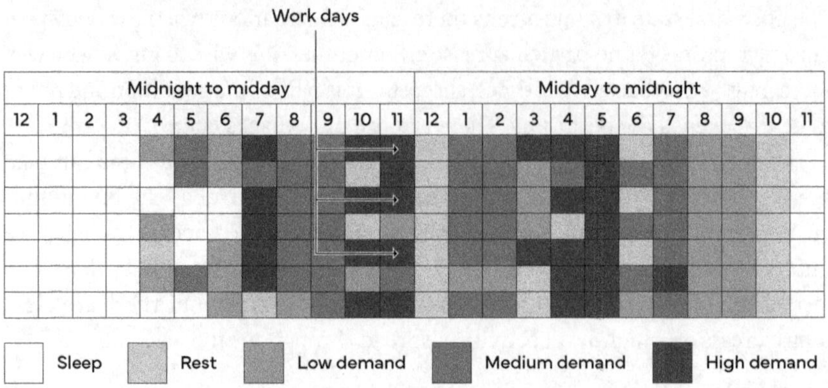

Figure 14.6 Liz's diary with adapted work, sleep management and rest breaks

How we engage in an activity: Feeling tone

Buddhist psychology and practice identifies that 'feeling tone'; in other words, how we feel about what we feel or perceive 'is one of the five essential factors acting together with embodiment and environment in any moment: contact, feeling tone, perception, attention, and intention to act' (Williams et al. 2022). Mindfulness courses touch on this through the programme: in the third session, participants are invited to consider how pleasant events feel and unpack what a pleasant experience means in terms of emotion, sensation, embodiment, thoughts and urges to act; in the fourth session, unpleasant events are explored in a similar way. Learning to respond rather than react or act according to habitual patterns of reactivity is an important aspect of mindfulness. It could also be useful for those having to scrutinize their energy and make difficult choices.

The session on nurturing and depleting activity develops this further. We have taken the hot-air balloon metaphor (Figure 14.7) as this is an embodied way to approach it – What lifts me, fills me up like a balloon? And what drags me down like heavy sandbags? Usually, someone identifies that mindfulness is the whole balloon, that life both lifts and drags down, and that we can make choices by increasing the flame that heats the air.

'Energy' components of an activity are likely to be affected by how we feel, and it could be very useful to be able to identify that there are parts of my experience I like, parts I don't, and parts I was not even aware of and perhaps had the overriding feeling of boredom. Personally, I know that if I have a day or two where I do more administrative tasks than clinical work I do not feel very happy; if I don't get outside at the weekend, I can feel uptight and grumpy. For some, it can be helpful to record how they are responding to activity, as, for example, in Table 14.1.

What lifts me?

Sunshine	Friendship
Standing up for myself	Conversation
Achieving	Being understood
something/taking	Sharing
action	Connecting
Being in nature	with people and
Fresh air	environment
Music	Choice
Challenging myself	Mastery

What drags me down?

The news…	Life admin
Arguments	Reading above my baseline
Housework	Forms
Overthinking past situations or	Dealing with energy companies
encounters	Being sick – aware of workload building
Strong emotions – of any flavour	
Managing appointments	

Figure 14.7 Hot-air balloon of life (adapted from the Bangor Teacher Training Retreat 2)

Table 14.1 Activities: Feelings

Time	Activity	Feelings about activity
7.30	Got up, showered	Neutral/pleasant
8.30	Checked email	Stressed/unpleasant
9.30	Read paper	Neutral
11.00	Walked to shop	Pleasant

This record can be combined with the high-, medium- and low-energy requirements, and some useful information can emerge. In Table 14.2, the quality or the 'tone' of the two medium-level activities is different, and the high-level activity is regarded as pleasant. This could then affect my understanding of how I felt later in the day, and perhaps might change how I schedule or approach the task. It can be nuanced further by considering the type of activity, is it predominantly mental, physical or emotional activity? Would this change how I planned my day? (Table 14.3).

Table 14.2 Activities: High, medium and low

Time	Activity	High, medium, low	Feelings about activity
7.30	Got up, showered	M	Neutral/pleasant
8.30	Checked email	M	Stressed/unpleasant
9.30	Read paper	L	Neutral
11.00	Walked to shop	H	Pleasant

Table 14.3 Activities: Mental, physical and emotional

Time	Activity	Mental, physical, emotional	High, medium, low	Feelings about activity
7.30	Got up, showered	P	M	Neutral/pleasant
8.30	Checked email	M/E	M	Stressed/unpleasant
9.30	Read paper	M	L	Neutral
11.00	Walked to shop	P	H	Pleasant

As an example, if I've been working at a computer all day, is watching TV (another screen) in the evening really a light activity or a rest? It may well be a light activity in some circumstances, but in this context, the balance of type of activity is skewed to (physically) sitting and (sensory) looking at a screen and (cognitive) taking in information. Do I need to find something else that uses different modalities, perhaps more physical and mentally simplified; for example, go for a short walk, stroke the cat, make a cake, deadhead flowers, see a friend? There is no right way to do this; personal preferences are very important here, as some people seem to find colouring, jigsaws and knitting soothing, I don't!

Texture or flavour of activity

The texture, flavour or quality of an activity, the way that we engage with it and how we feel when we are occupied can vary hugely. As discussed in chapter 8, Gilbert's work on emotional regulation systems that broadly clusters our responses into three systems, Drive, Threat/protection and Soothing/connecting (Gilbert 2020; Gilbert and Choden 2013), can be a helpful way to consider this texture when carrying out an activity.

If we imagine doing any activity at all, let's say chopping a tomato for a salad, in a soothing way we might be listening to music, taking in the colour, smell and texture of the tomato and have no particular time to get it done. In Drive we might be chopping it in a particular way (slices or quarters or diced…) for a certain recipe we are following and also logging it in a food diary. In Threat/ protection mode we might be taking out our stress of the day imagining we are stabbing someone or perhaps having a heated discussion at the same time and feeling generally wound up. In this mode, we could also decide we cannot be bothered to chop the tomato and give up completely.

Self-assessment – which system am I in?

As part of activity analysis this exercise can be used to identify how we move through the systems.

Keep a note of what you do in a day and note which system you are in (Table 14.4).

Table 14.4 Activities: Emotional systems

Activity	Emotional system
Wake up and make tea	Soothing–Drive
Realize I'm late and kids aren't up	Threat–Drive
Drive to work	Drive
Can't find a parking space (and I'm late)	Threat
Colleague makes me a coffee and tells me a funny story	Soothing
Computer breaks down	Threat
Go home	Drive
Traffic jam	Threat
Drink wine	Threat/protection

How do you think the person felt at the end of this day?

If you did this for yourself, can you spot a pattern? Which systems are you mainly in? How do they link, e.g. do you go from Threat to Drive to Threat?

Do the routines support the intentions of the day and the way one wishes to live? Are you able to engage and participate in your chosen occupations?

Can you improve balance by going from Threat to Soothing? And appreciate Drive and Soothing by paying attention and appreciating those states?

The same day is shown in Table 14.5 with more options. Notice: pausing, choice of activity, connection to wider social experience, values and appreciation of self, others and the environment.

Table 14.5 Activities: Emotional systems with more options

Activity	Emotional system
Wake up and make tea	Soothing–Drive
Realize I'm late and kids aren't up	Threat–Drive
Pause – notice they have now got up, other parent is on it and it is going to be OK, kiss kids goodbye	(Soothing)
Drive to work	Drive
Listen to music or story	(Soothing)
Can't find a parking space (and I'm late)	Threat
Therapeutic swearing! Then tell myself I'm doing as best I can. Breathe; notice the sky. Text supportive colleague.	(Soothing)

cont.

Activity	Emotional system
Colleague makes me a coffee and tells me a funny story	Soothing
Feel gratitude for colleague and notice I'm smiling	(Enhanced Soothing/connection)
Computer breaks down	Threat
Notice I'm feeling tense; take some deep breaths and pause while I decide what to do	(Soothing/Drive)
Contact the IT dept who identify it is a system error, arrange for the dept system to be fixed	(Drive)
Appreciate the IT consultant's help	(Soothing/connection)
Go home	Drive
Traffic jam	Threat
Notice my body response – it's not my fault, my body does this because it's trying to protect me; realize I can't do anything about it; breathe; notice what's outside the car; listen to comedy on the radio	(Soothing)
Drink wine	Threat/protection
Turn that into soothing pleasure – share with a friend (either in person or on phone/Skype) or listen to music and make sure I eat and drink water too and only have one or two glasses	(Soothing/connection)

How do you think the person felt at the end of this day?

Note that switching between systems doesn't take any more time or effort. The key is to be aware and compassionate and have a variety of resources, recalling that Soothing includes reaching out to others, and this can be a direct way to reduce feelings of Threat.

Switching between types of activity and system

Returning to the mechanisms of mindfulness (Shapiro et al. 2006), after becoming aware, we can consider our intention, place attention, and tend to our attitude. In fatigue management this can add to awareness of the type of activity one is doing:

- Is it predominantly physical or mental activity?
- Is it something I must do or want to do?
- Have I been in Threat mode and need to soothe before I go on to the next thing?
- Have I been in Drive mode and need to stop and rest and appreciate what I have achieved and/or enjoyed?

- Have I been relaxing and engaging in gentle activity for a while and need to get some jobs done that will give me a sense of satisfaction?
- Can I approach my tasks in a way that will maintain Drive but not overdo it so that I don't end up fatigued and in pain and in Threat mode? This may mean planning and prioritizing both the activity and the rest required and balancing high- and low-level activity over a period of time.

Bringing mindfulness to setbacks

A setback is when there is a flare-up of symptoms that leads to a period of time when the normal level of activity is not achievable. This is a more prolonged period of lowered activity than the boom-and-bust cycle of post-exertional symptom exacerbation that many navigate over a day, week or month. It can be a very difficult time as an individual may have been managing for a while but then becomes demoralized as their efforts to get better are not paying off.

Having setbacks is a distinct experience that is an inevitable part of living with fatiguing and pain conditions. They can come about for a number of reasons, including having another illness or injury, a period of extra activity, and stressful or difficult events; but pleasurable and exciting events can also take their toll, as can an unexpected event, and so on. A period of poor sleep can also have an impact. Or it could be a change in circumstances causing symptoms to flare up. Sometimes, it can feel that they come out of the blue, and it can particularly feel like this if management has been going well for a while and life is feeling under control...and then it changes. Perhaps too there is a subtle effect of things going on in the world that takes its toll (Coakley and Knops 2022).

Managing setbacks is part of living with a health condition. Having a plan to deal with them and, if possible, spot them upstream is a skill people need to develop. Without this, there can be a fear that gains made will be lost and that progress means constant improvement which can be put off course by the challenges of life. Having some strategies in place can hugely increase confidence and a sense of control over life's challenges.

'The pit'

The pit is a metaphor for capturing what we do to manage life when things are OK and then what happens when things get tricky – a way of mindfully managing setbacks (Figure 14.8). It comes from the expression of 'being in the pits'. This metaphor has long been used in the Bristol service pain management and ME/CFS teams.

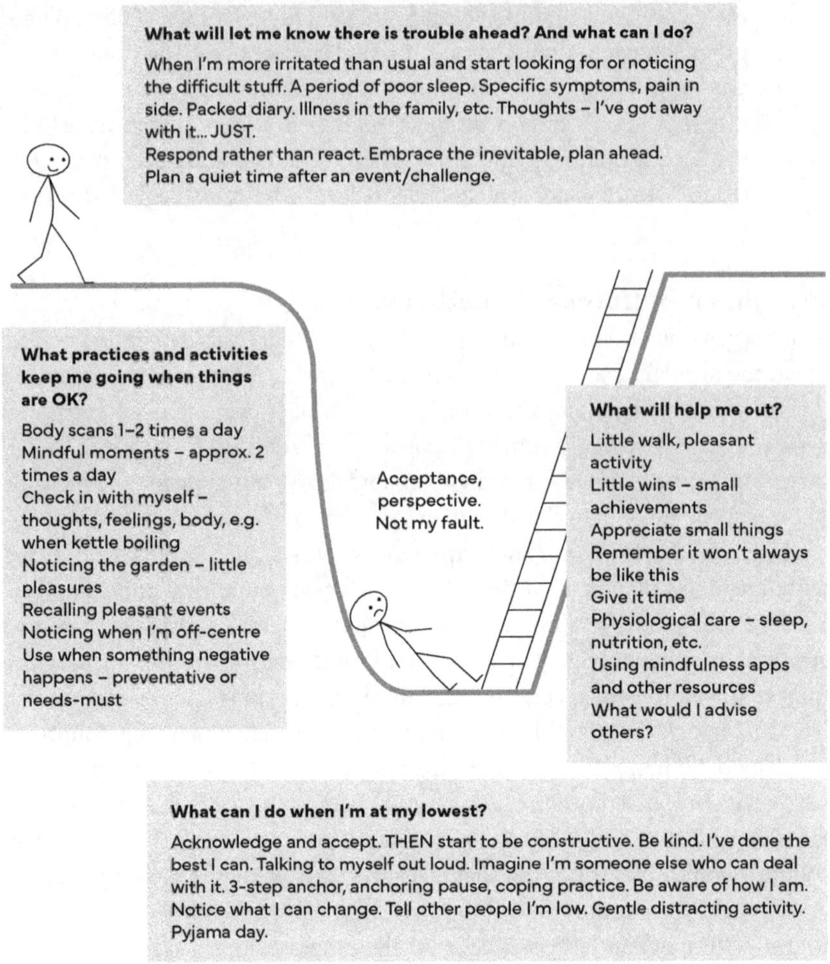

Figure 14.8 Mindfully managing setbacks – examples

The image of walking along through some countryside is fleshed out by considering that the ground isn't going to be smooth, there will be small ups and downs, and having some ways of self-managing and regular practices to support day-to-day living can be very useful. If this was an actual pit in the countryside, in the UK there would most likely be a sign saying 'Pit ahead, take care'. This metaphor is used to discuss the signs of a setback looming. There can be symptoms; however, these are likely to be early signs we are tumbling into the pit, so this gives an opportunity to differentiate between symptoms and what may lead to setback. Then thinking about what action needs to be taken to avoid falling in the pit or perhaps to find a way out of it. Participants report that over the time of practising and working with this, they can come out of setbacks much faster and not go so deep.

How people are when they are at the bottom of the pit is important. Fighting it and pushing and feeling hopeless and disempowered is likened to digging it deeper. Keeping going with the analogy, often it is impossible to stop setbacks but maybe we can get out the crash mats and have some tools ready to help. Having a ladder ready to get out is part of an individual self-care plan, and this gives space to consider what needs to be prepared in advance, including a reminder of what to do, as coming up with ideas when one is in the pit is extremely difficult. The previous work with the systems and Being and Doing mind is useful as people recognize they will be in Threat and it is very difficult to come up with a Soothing or appropriate Drive response at that point.

Mindfulness offers several things here:

- Regular practices to manage the day-to-day that has its ups and downs but with prioritizing planning and pacing activity, having regular rests and a mindfulness practice that allows rest, observation and reflection and an opportunity to notice the pleasant as well as the unpleasant. Things can feel manageable and life can open up with this new way of doing things.
- When setbacks do arise, the ability to notice how one feels but also the context for that. Someone described it as being a torch they could use to light up the pit to see what it consisted of, where it came from and, most importantly, where the ladder was to get out.
- Self-care and compassion rather than recrimination and spiralling thinking when one is in the pits, or at least, reducing the time in challenging self-talk and unhelpful actions (and forgiving oneself when we spot that we have not been helping ourselves).
- An understanding that things change over time. Sometimes that is all that is needed, and mindfulness can help us see how things can change, moment by moment.
- The attitudinal foundations, including patience, curiosity, trust, acceptance, non-judging, non-striving and letting go.
- An opportunity for reflection and also compassion for oneself. The cause could be contracting another illness, a period of insomnia, a period of stress or a time of increased activity because there was a reduction in symptoms. The symptoms that herald the setback could be sore throats, feeling worse in the mornings, some generalized aching. Participants note that this often means they can end up doing more at this point because they 'know what's coming'.

Wider participation

The model of human occupation (Figure 14.9), an occupational therapy model (Kielhofner 2002), looks at wider factors, such as the human and physical context, our values, goals and motivations, and the habits and roles we occupy, as well as the skills that can support our self-management and engagement in occupations (that is, any activity we want to do or must do). Mindfulness itself is an occupation – it is skill-based, and in the process of learning it we use particular skills, but we also need the intention (or volition) to both practise and apply the skills in different contexts. The habits and roles we occupy will support or challenge our capacity to embed a mindfulness-based approach, which in this model then enables an increased potential for adaptation and competency in this new way of being.

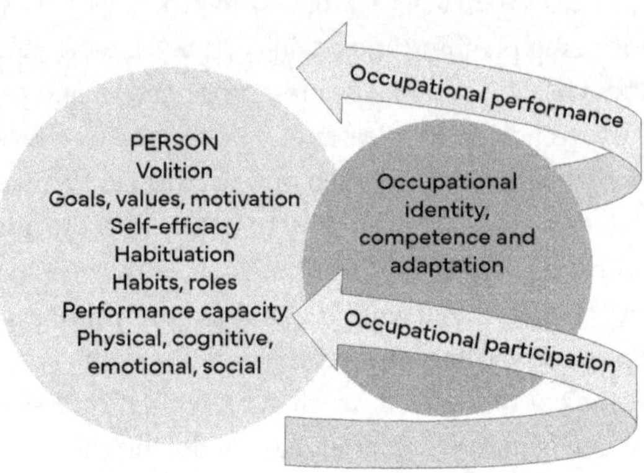

Figure 14.9 Model of human occupation (adapted from Parkinson, Forsyth and Kielhofner 2004)

By increasing occupational participation, the Soothing system is enhanced, as connection with others is part of this system. Being part of the tribe is an aspect of humanity that underlies many of our behaviours; feeling outside of the tribe leaves us vulnerable and threatened. Illness that creates barriers to participation enlivens the Threat/protection response. By connecting through valued occupations, both Drive and Soothing are accessed. Helping people find a way to do things is practical, but additionally being able to do what matters most to us is satisfying and can lead to a greater sense of well-being (Durocher, Gibson and Rappolt 2014; Hocking, Townsend and Mace 2021).

Returning to the examples at the beginning of the chapter, Sindra and Carlos adapted their activity in a way that increased their participation both socially *and* within their chosen occupations. If they had remained fixed on doing things as they always had done, the net result could have been decreasing participation and competency (Taylor et al. 2003).

Applying and extending the approach, including participation in the workplace

As an illustration, we'll look at the example of Jane. Jane worked in the NHS and had glandular fever five years ago and was admitted with sepsis. She took eight months off work to recover, gradually improved and went back to work on a phased return. She reduced to part-time hours and managed for a while, but things became harder. After six months, she was off work again for four months, went back to even fewer hours and started with a phased return. This lasted for 18 months before being signed off again after several episodes of sickness relating to fatigue. By now, her mood dropped and she was referred to the ME/CFS service and embarked on an activity-management programme with support from an occupational therapist (OT) and psychologist. She then did the mindfulness-based programme and felt she made good progress, so returned to work again. The same thing happened, she went off work, and she contacted the mindfulness teacher/OT as she was aware she was struggling to implement what worked at home into her work life, despite adjustments.

In the sessions, we reflected on what did work. She was able to use the breath to pause and rest; she prioritized activity at home and engaged in physical activity in a new way. She had previously been very sporty and competitive with herself as well as others. One of her previous strategies had been to get rid of the Fitbit that gave her speed and time and focus on enjoying a walk, using skills from the mindfulness programme. At home, she could pace what she did with her partner and grandchildren and it worked out OK, they understood.

We analysed what happened at work, and Jane identified that she not only liked her job, but wanted to be thought well of in her team and was often the first to volunteer to take on jobs, and if they were to be shared out, she routinely would do more. She rarely took breaks and would frequently stay late.

We contrasted her strategies at home to how she was working, and she reflected: 'It's like I walk into work and I forget who I am now; I go back to how I have always worked.' We reflected on what might help:

- Prioritizing and planning tasks, including location as the workplace was very large.
- Setting a goal, e.g. one appointment per session.
- A quiet place to write up notes – a work laptop could be provided.
- Finding places to pause and rest and scheduling smaller and longer breaks.
- Some work from home, e.g. online training, reports, etc.
- Regular supervision to agree workloads.
- Phased return increase to be in phases completed and managed rather than set dates with very low starting hours.

- Clear rest days when not in work.

Some of the barriers to this were external – the shortage of staff due to sickness and changes during the pandemic meant there were additional complications. This stressed the rest of the team who were often working longer hours and without breaks.

The support at work was apparent – her manager and supervisor agreed with the above plan and were aware of Jane's tendencies to want to support her colleagues and be very involved. We all agreed that while starting at home was an idea, the real challenge would be when she stepped into the hospital and went into 'work role'.

How can mindfulness-based therapy support this situation? Jane came up with the following:

- Noticing the specifics of my situation and where things are easier or more challenging.
- Noticing that I have home and work roles – I can see that I am still me when I do things differently in my sports and home life; I have accepted that, but I don't accept the changes I need to make at work. The changes at work felt more charged.
- Reperceiving the situation – 'there are many ways to do my work'.

We looked at developing a new way of working bearing in mind awareness of these challenges. Using an inquiry-based approach, we devised some experiments and developed themes, including watching colleagues with different working styles – some did take breaks and would only take on things they knew they could do; getting permission from managers and supervisors to work in this 'new way'; agreeing it was an acceptable way to work. Other new ways of working and thinking about work included:

- Noting hooks to particular action; for example, wanting to take on more when Jane could see stressed colleagues. Noticing the urge to step in. But also remembering her plan of action using baselines and breaks was not taking her away from work, rather it meant she was able to work more reliably.

  Seeing triggers to particular reactions as 'hooks' was a more active metaphor than a 'trigger' that sets us off, but there is nothing in that metaphor that can be worked with: a hook can be unhooked and the process of 'hooking' can be slower and perhaps spotted, whereas a 'trigger' sets off a very fast bullet. Hooking also enables a choice: I can perhaps choose where I am hooking myself.

- What's important here? 'I am more helpful going in and doing something small than not being there.' This was uncomfortable, but being clear about what was important helped, as did the acknowledgement that this was not easy – the urges will come, can I turn towards them, take care of myself? Step back, see the bigger picture?
- What is the underlying motivation? And what are the facts that this is based upon? Ultimately, there needed to be a bigger motivation than it being better for her and her colleagues in the long run. Clarifying and being explicit about the importance of work to her not only profession-ally but financially, she articulated that she wanted to work so she would have a reasonable pension and needed to do another 1.5 years at this level. Pushing herself and going off sick again could have implications going forward and affect her partner and their plans.

  We agreed that recalling the need to remain in work, and therefore the need to work in a sustainable way, may be useful. However, after some research, she and her partner also acknowledged that if a different out-come arose and she did have to leave work, then they would be able to deal with it, which reduced the underlying feeling of stress and drive and urgency around work.

Some further work was done on identifying the longstanding patterns of working that predated the glandular fever and were driving her to work above what she could sustain. We used preparatory visualization to explore an ideal day at work and reinforce taking breaks, resting and sticking to her work plan, and used mindfulness to become aware that even when the day was imagined there were hooks and pitfalls that she could then notice and manage proactively when she was in situ.

After six months working through the pandemic and the pressure of win-ter in the NHS, Jane has taken retirement and is positive about her life going forward. The mindfulness-based approach meant she had skills and resources to ground herself and look at what was going on and make decisions based on the reality of the situation rather than longstanding patterns of pushing and needing to be 'useful'.

SUMMARY

- Mindful activity is part of learning mindfulness; however, we are missing the point of the practice if the focus is only on how we do the practice and having discrete mindful moments.

- Living with a health condition is complex, and mindful awareness offers a way to observe what is going on and find choice points.
- Having ways of analysing the demands of activity, the feeling tone (like/dislike/neutral) and the emotional texture of activity can support self-management.
- Observing patterns of levels of activity but also type of activity and being aware of personal references, balance, goals, values and intentions can feel overwhelming but if done in stages and with support can increase the capacity to manage and participate in activity as well as social situations which are important elements of health.

Chapter 15

Rest – What It Is and How We Do It

- Challenge of rest when living with fatigue
- Defining rest
- Rest in action and for action
- A mindfulness approach to rest

Meditation is seen often as a restful thing to do; however, as many find, stopping and focusing the mind is often not restful. There are often suggestions given to stay awake, 'fall awake' (Kabat-Zinn 2013) through attention, keeping the eyes open, raising a hand and other strategies that are perhaps not restful and point to a different intention. Claudia Hammond's book *The Art of Rest* (2019) describes a large study on rest by the Wellcome Foundation (Hammond and Lewis 2016) and identifies that while mindfulness meditation is seen by some to be rest it does come 10th in the top 10 strategies people use. This is to me unsurprising (perhaps surprising it makes the top 10!) as mindfulness is of itself not intended to do anything apart from bring a gentle awareness and curiosity with a light intention. Hammond's prescription for rest is in in fact imbued with mindfulness, and our experience is that mindfulness can support rest, albeit not necessarily restful of itself.

The use of rest and relaxation techniques can be very important, but this is not easy work. A mindfulness-based approach can support both understanding the experience of rest and how that may have changed for an individual and develop embodied practices to support rest. This mindfulness programme folds in rest and pauses and overtly looks at ways to stop, pause and rest with a health condition that can find rest extremely uncomfortable. This chapter will consider what rest is, the challenges of resting and the role a mindfulness-based approach can play in supporting rest when living with a fluctuating condition.

Many of the people I meet in the clinic appear full of life and energy; however, we know from the depleted and painful few days that often soon follow that this is usually not a constant state. Rest and sleep not only don't give relief from exhaustion, they are both difficult and uncomfortable to the point it can be easier to keep pushing and then collapse and get up again when possible – 'keep going until I drop'. We tend to meet people when this strategy is no longer working and the result is often a net reduction in activity, and the return to activity after a 'crash' lowers and lowers over time creating more struggle and in many cases a significant impact on life.

Why can't I rest?

These are some observations, from discussions with many patients about their experiences, on what it can feel like to stop and 'rest' when in reality we become increasingly aware of the stress reaction in the body and mind. Mindfulness invites us to feel this, notice and act compassionately. In this case, I needed to keep moving, slowly, feel the pain and then gradually bring myself to rest.

> 'The urge to keep going was compelling.'
> 'Stopping, tingling, stinging awareness of perpetual motion.'
> 'Stopping physically in terms of moving or getting anywhere looks like I'm at rest, but aware of a neurological zinging ringing whizzing in my brain and through the body. Mind racing, heart beating, whirring, whooshing in my ears. Limbs tensing; jaw clenching.'
> 'Familiar patterns of holding on, literally by the skin of my teeth...'
> 'Not rest.'
> 'More effort than moving.'
> 'Maximal awareness of sound, light, tactile sense.'
> 'Slightest movement brings relief yet a sense of needing to begin to stop again...'

The alarm-system model (see chapter 3) is useful for understanding this; if we see the fatigue and symptoms as being caused by an overactive protective system that does not stop and in fact responds to distress, exertion, challenge with more effort, then we are not in the state of 'rest and digest' (parasympathetic nervous system activation) or healing. The state people experience is more a state of collapse, which in turn generates more protective (sympathetic and immune) activation.

Additionally, a restful state is not achieved by ordering oneself to rest, it needs to be 'felt' into, 'allowed' in much the same way we 'fall' asleep; we can create the conditions for rest and sleep to happen, but we cannot command ourselves to rest or sleep.

The three emotional regulation systems (see chapter 8) are useful here. Rest will be an element of the Soothing system, so is timeless, goalless, connected, gentle and absorbing. It can be supported by the satisfaction obtained through the Drive system, and rest can allow us to appreciate what we can achieve in Drive, as well as the way the Threat system is inhibited.

The how, when and where of rest – as well as what

Let's start with what... According to the online dictionary etymonine.com, the word *rest* has various etymologies. In Old English *ræste* or *reste* means a bed or a couch, intermission of labour, mental peace, a state of quiet or repose. In Old Saxon it means a burial place, and in Old German and in Norse it meant a league of miles (after which one stopped and rested). Later meanings were rests in music (16th century) and also a remainder, from what has been separated out – 'the rest'. The expression 'rest up' (in order to gain strength) is later still (19th century).

The Cambridge Dictionary has three main categories of contemporary definitions of rest with different underlying meanings:

1. recovery, strength, support
2. steadiness, dependability
3. dead, not working, left out, set aside, stopped.

It seems we use this little word to mean many things. Someone who sees resting as recovery, steadiness and a means of dependable support is likely to have a different experience to one who sees the experience of resting as being left out, stopping and ultimately dying. Awareness of what the word means in the context of perhaps having to rest due to a health problem can be useful. If my dependability and steadiness comes from being present all the time and working hard and being useful, then resting could feel like I'm left out, unreliable and the end of my involvement in a meaningful, useful or gainful way. Taken further, hard work is embedded in Western culture through the Protestant work ethic, which at its basis sees hard work as being godly, and loafing and slothfulness as serving the devil. How we perceive rest individually and within our families and upbringing (consciously and unconsciously) is crucial to how we might perceive rest.

Mindful awareness of what rest can mean to individuals can be very helpful. We may very well not have an overt understanding that resting means we are left out and morally bankrupt, but by tapping in to how it feels, and what that might mean, can be enlightening. Rhonda Knight describes her experience as a nurse: 'We never stopped, not even to go to the loo; I realize that part of the training was to override my feelings, as the patients and the needs of the ward were the most important thing.'

When Rhonda started the course, she struggled to connect or feel her body at all; I recall sitting with her and inviting her to feel into the back of the chair, to feel where the chair touched her, and she responded, 'Nope, nothing at all.' With this background, it is easy to see how rest is not only not seen as not important but has no benefit or use, and also how some can develop the ability to push on despite significant symptoms and then need to stop for prolonged periods of time. And how painful that is, if in your bones stopping feels so wrong, and yet we are advised to 'just rest'.

The art of rest

Rest can mean many things to many people, and is an art rather than a 'technique' or a tool. It will vary over time and hugely from person to person. Claudia Hammond (2019, p.251) identifies six ingredients for rest:

- Taking a break from other people
- Resting your mind as well as your body
- Exerting your body in order to rest your mind
- Being distracted from your worries
- Allowing your mind to wander
- Giving yourself permission not to achieve anything in particular.

How these ingredients are mixed is going to vary from person to person. For many of us, our interests and passions are a source of joy and nourishment, as well as enabling us to rest, as we are engaged in something entirely for its own pleasure and can allow our mind to gently wander, rest our minds, be released from our worries and others.

The challenge of rest

For those living with a health condition, tried and tested routines and ways of doing things can be severely disrupted; this can be confusing as well as distressing as the above ingredients can feel out of reach. This can lead to activities that were used to balance out daily stress, exerting the body in order to rest the mind and add to a sense of well-being becoming no longer available. The following examples are of people where this significantly affected their ability to rest and restore:

- Dinesh: 'I used to climb mountains and wild camp to get away from everything.'
- Sally: 'I used to run 3k every day and 10k at the weekends. This kept me sane, rested my mind and I was away from everyone. Planning routes was also enjoyable and absorbing.'
- Aika: 'I loved my allotment, just being there gave me a sense of peace.'

- Jenny: 'I liked meeting friends to wild swim and walk, I felt connected to nature and safe with my friends.'

All of them used their loved activity and found the memories and the planning of it gave moments of calm and pleasure and an escape from the day-to-day, but now:

- Dinesh can only walk for ten minutes a day and becomes breathless going up hills or steps.
- Sally can only go out in a wheelchair.
- Aika can manage home and her garden but not the allotment.
- Jenny can socialize at home for only about two hours. She's lost touch with a lot of her friends.

The sense of loss is huge, and though we know that many things can return in some form, it takes a long time, years. While writing this, Sarah Nearney sent me a photo sent from the ski slopes: '...here for the first time in eight years; no black runs, spa days instead; but I'm here and on skis doing the mountain meditation with the Eiger!' Others will not return to strenuous activity but find new ways of being:

- Dinesh remains hopeful, is gradually increasing his walking ability, but this is slow, and he is also mourning his old self and having additional support for his mental health.
- Sally found Buddhist meditation after the mindfulness course and has developed her practice and interest with a meditation group and retreats often in beautiful locations.
- Aika: 'I am learning to paint the flowers and birds in my garden.'
- Jenny: 'I have set up an Instagram account of micro-photography and spend hours absorbed in the detail of plants and insects and enjoy the appreciative feedback I receive.'

How to rest

If we analyse rest as an activity, rest is considered to be between sleep and low-level activity, which are each on their own continuums (Figure 15.1). We make the distinction that rest is different to both sleep and light activity as this is an important part of managing fatigue and learning the art of rest. Sleep for many people we see is not restful and needs its own management; light activity can be pleasant and nourishing but is not the same as rest. Being able to distinguish the three and knowing when one is becoming the other can be a useful part of self-management.

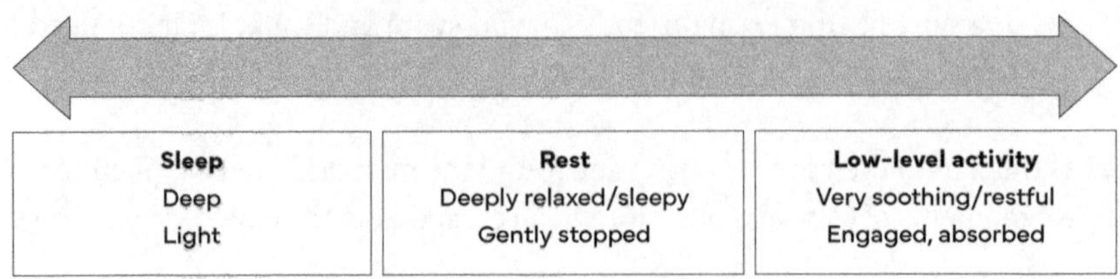

Figure 15.1 Sleep–Rest–Activity continuums

> Sitting on the sofa wrapped up in a blanket listening to an audio book can be a low-level restful activity that leads me to feel rested and perhaps drowsy, and I have a few moments of light sleep at the end of the chapter. Listening to the book is an activity, rest is the drowsiness, and while there is sleep, a few moments of light sleep can still be considered rest as that won't affect night-time sleep (a 20-minute power nap can be considered a rest). Whereas sitting on the sofa watching TV after work, falling asleep can be unpleasant; it is more a shutting down than a rest, a state of collapse, and will also potentially disrupt my night-time sleep.

It can be helpful to distinguish stages of rest. David Whyte (2019) describes five phases that I paraphrase here:

1. Stopping what or how we are doing something
2. Coming home to the body
3. Arriving (finding a sense of healing)
4. Resting in the breath (feeling rest as an exchange of give and take)
5. Readiness to return to the world.

...we are rested when we let things alone and let ourselves alone, to do what we do best, breathe as the body intended us to breathe, to walk as we were meant to walk, to live with the rhythm of a house and home... When we give and take in an easy foundational way, we are closest to the authentic self, and closest to that self when we are most rested. (Whyte 2019, p.182)

In the boom-and-bust cycle, the collapse in the bust is not rest, it is recovery from the fight/flight response being activated, and the system is going into a state of retreat. Many of us do need periods of recovery, but this needs to be identified and cared for, and distinguished from rest. The Drive and Soothing modes allow us this as we enjoy the buzz for achieving, enjoying and connecting and then soothe with appreciating, acknowledging and nurturing. There is some evidence that focusing on good things and bringing mindful presence to what is 'good' in the moment positively affects well-being (e.g. Hanson et al. 2021).

The scholar and Buddhist teacher Thich Nhat Hanh talks of 'being peace', which is an active connection to a state that is available to all. Seeing it in this way, I concur with David Whyte: resting is not always while one is still, 'we can be rested while putting together an elaborate meal for an arriving crowd, whilst climbing the highest mountain or sitting at home surrounded by the chaos is a living family' (Whyte 2019). Being able to access this opens up opportunities and reduces fear:

- Janet: 'I wanted to travel, I didn't feel I could, I didn't know how to begin, so one day I just went to the train station, I used the pauses to check in with myself, shake off additional tension; noticed what was OK and asked for help. I was helped onto the train by station staff, was comfortable and did my practice on the train. I did it, I went on a journey, it was exciting and I enjoyed it, and I did need to rest once I got home. I will do it again.'
- Heather: 'I can't take breaks at work, it feels wrong as a nurse to do so and makes me feel more stressed.' Instead, we looked at where she got fulfilment from her job (being with patients) and she rested in that, was very present, feeling her feet on the floor, connecting to her breath, and after each patient when she was washing her hands, she took in what she was doing. She also noticed when she was being knocked off centre during work, and actively grounded herself, noticed what was going on and made considered choices about what to do next rather than reacting and pushing through. 'If I do this throughout the day, I've noticed I'm not so exhausted at the end of the day.'

These reported examples of 'resting in action' are linked to what is important to each person; in Janet's case it was to travel, in Heather's it was to work as a nurse and be present for her patients. In both cases, withdrawal to rest would have been a 'recovery' from a state of pushing. By accessing a sense of peace within the valued activity they are engaged within, they are able to find nourishment and a sense of uplift during the activity that seems to be accumulative; as Heather says: 'I'm not so exhausted at the end of the day.' Theoretically this suggests that the system is less wound up and may mean people can rest more effectively when they eventually have a longer break.

Mindfulness and resting

Mindfulness practice is not a rest *per se*, but it can be. It is perhaps better to see it as a process and an approach that can help us access a restful state that is within us all. As we have seen, rest is many things. In the mindfulness programme, we introduce the practices in a way that they can be a rest as well as mindfulness of resting.

Stopping

Learning to stop and rest the body in a way that does actually rest is an art and practice of itself. This is distinct from taking a break, being distracted and exerting the body in order to rest the mind as described in Hammond's (2019) prescription for rest. The home practice is an invitation to stop. However, the guided practices can only be done on purpose and are more pleasant if one has not overdone things beforehand. An unwinding is encouraged, through finding the floor and letting the body drop so the centre of gravity is lowered, as Vidyamala Burch in the Breathworks programme (Burch and Penman 2013) describes in the gorgeous practice of 'giving in to gravity' and adapted here:

> Let the furniture you are sitting or lying on take your weight; let the floor below take your weight and then feel yourself supported by the building you are in; all the way down through the foundations of the building to the earth below. Let the earth take your weight. Then make yourself a little more comfortable, letting the body move in order to allow this.

This practice on its own is a rest and can be used in any situation. We start all our practices with this for several reasons: repetition means the body then gets accustomed to 'dropping and feeling support' so a new habit is developed as well as a skill; in doing this, you don't have to get your mind on board, you let your body lead the way. The guidance is direct ('Drop your weight') rather than curious about how you do it, or assuming that one can stop; it directs the individual to take a particular action, and a slight shift in weight can be noticed as one purposely lets oneself drop into the furniture and floor. It may take practice, but along with the direction to 'make yourself a little more comfortable' our feedback shows that most can find a way to do this and continue this practice in daily life long after the course has finished. The connection with furniture and the floor and the sensations of connection can support people who have an element of trauma (Treleaven 2018). In subsequent practices, there is an invitation to repeatedly return to the sense of physical connection with the earth and tangible sensation and to move as required to make oneself more comfortable.

> From this dropped, and possibly heavy, grounded place, become aware of the height of you, rising up through the torso, the spine, finding a sense of height and space in the centre of the body. Maintain a sense of the ground as well as the height. Feeling up through the body to the top of the head. Sense of uplift.

Let the shoulders move, perhaps dropping and rotating backwards; hands softening; belly releasing; jaw gently dropping.

More directions, encouraging a sense of action once we have stopped and dropped. The movement upwards can be literally uplifting for mood and bring a sense of energy and well-being. This movement perhaps heralds Whyte's 5th element of rest, readiness to return to the world, the possibility of this being seeded early in the practice. However, for now we are still stopping and perhaps aware of pain, tension and unease:

Scan through the body and invite any additional, tensing, holding or gripping to release if it can. If it cannot, allow it to be there and take care of yourself as best you can.

This is another direct instruction, not asking us to relax but to let go, if possible, of additional tension that may not be required right now. And if we can't, then to let it be but take care of ourselves perhaps through movement, diverted attention, soothing self-talk or just letting it be amidst all the other sensations. Noticing where this additional tension can be released is reinforcing and empowering:

'I didn't know I was so tight in my legs; by letting them drop and shift, the tension shifted significantly.'

'My neck is sore and tight but I realized I was holding my hands very tightly; I let them open and stretch.'

By letting the sensations we don't like and cannot do anything about be there, but perhaps be amidst something else that may be OK, and asking 'What do I need to take care of myself?', we are allowing a compassionate and forgiving response to be possible. To this end, we encourage people to make changes in posture at any point – maybe I am sitting and need to be lying or standing, maybe I need to roll onto my side. This may help, or we realize that it cannot be changed for now. So how do I take care of that? In the room sessions this also led to a conversation about not wanting to disturb others, which resulted in feedback that no one noticed or, if they did notice, they really didn't mind and were glad the other person was looking after themselves. And actually, it inspired someone else also to move.

The inquiry 'What do I need to do to take care of myself' can then move out of the group into how people take care of themselves within their own contexts and perhaps start to offer new ways of relating, describing their experience and asking for help.

Asking what is needed for care of oneself in the moment can make rest seem possible and expand the repertoire of what rest is.

Insight

Stopping, pausing, resting gives rise to a space where wisdom can develop. In the pause and the reflection, we can sometimes witness habitual mind and body patterns (e.g. when I stand up I grit my teeth; I must rest away from everyone else and not be in the way; I can only rest when the house is tidy), and question whether this is helpful for us at this point. In doing this, we can then create more helpful contexts for our ability to rest, realize when we are collapsing rather than resting and use other ways to manage this.

Compassion

This process of allowing ourselves to stop, to kindly witness our experience and open up to alternative ways of doing things is an act of compassion for ourselves, but often people start to realize that the more they are taking care of themselves the more available they can be to others. Letting ourselves see what is happening, our habits and instincts (both useful and not so helpful), can be either appreciated or forgiven, and from that perhaps other possibilities open out as we are ready to step back into giving and receiving in the wider world.

The four elements of stopping, resting, insight and compassion are interdependent; we can start at any one of them and find a way into the others. Figure 15.2 attempts to show this.

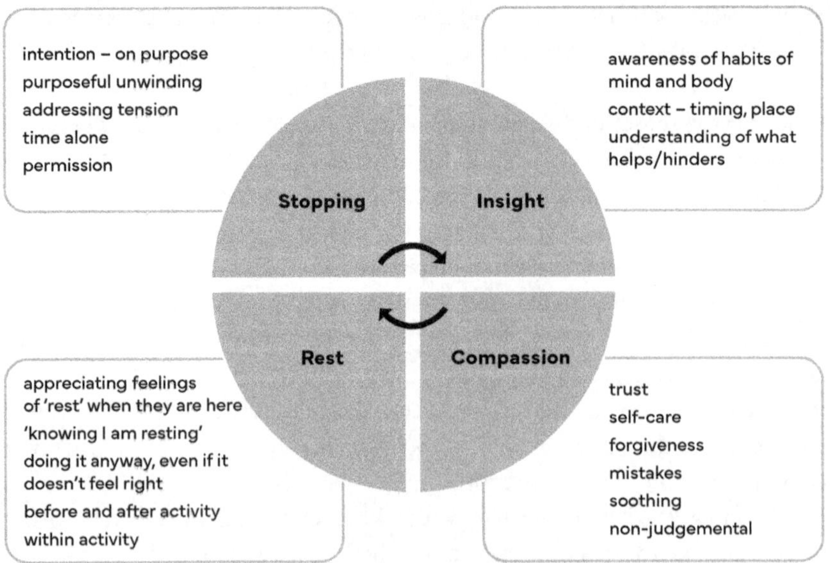

Figure 15.2 Components to enable rest

SUMMARY

- Resting is an art and can be very challenging when fatigued, when stopping means collapsing and perhaps increased awareness of tension, pain and exhaustion.
- People experiencing fatiguing health conditions may need to find wholly new ways of resting as previous strategies may no longer be available to them. This can in turn exacerbate feelings such as loss and guilt and lead to confusion, meaning it is even harder to rest.
- Mindfulness offers a way to insight into patterns of resting/not resting as well as practices that can enable rest.

The Mindfulness-Based Course for Fatigue

Part 4 shares the practical considerations for running the mindfulness courses, including assessment and follow-up and a week-by-week guide to the programme with a brief rationale. It needs to be borne in mind that while the sessions' intentions remain intact (usually), individual sessions might be adapted to any particular group's needs. Therefore, the outline of the course is very much a guide rather than a manual.

Rhonda Knight's reflection in chapter 18, 'Living with Fatigue: From Doing to Being', is a reflection on the programme as a participant. As she says in the beginning, she kept notes on the first course as a reflective learning journal and has added to them over the past ten years as she has continued to practise and share her practice with us.

As reiterated throughout this book, we have made changes of nuance and emphasis and the programme is very much based in the mindfulness-based cognitive therapy (Segal et al. 2013) and mindfulness-based stress reduction (Santorelli et al. 2017) programmes as taught at the Centre for Mindfulness Research and Practice at Bangor University.

In the final chapter we offer some thoughts on training and supervision and the role of clinician personal practice as well as clinical knowledge and understanding.

Chapter 16

Practical Considerations

	Recruitment and initial meetings
	Running courses in the room or on Zoom
	Need for administrative support
	Post-course follow-up

Recruitment to the courses

Over a year, approximately three afternoon and three morning courses run at two different hospital sites. People can be referred to the mindfulness-based programme from the pain management service, the ME/CFS service and the Long Covid programme. We expect people to have had some help within self-management (e.g. a pain-management programme) and understand the boom-and-bust cycle principles of pain and self-management, etc., as described in Part 1. The referring clinician's observations – diagnosis; what elements of the service have been accessed so far; and why mindfulness might be useful – all help in assessing suitability for the course.

Unless there is good reason for direct contact, we send the prospective participant information about the mindfulness programme and ask them to phone or email in if they would like to take it further, which builds on the self-management ethos of the department as participants can choose to opt in. There is a meeting to clarify how and whether a mindfulness-based approach may help, what experience people have had so far, and their understanding of mindfulness; and information about the intention and pragmatics of the course is shared. We have stopped calling the meeting or appointment an 'assessment' as feedback was that people felt they had to pass something, and that added an unnecessary edge to what was literally a meeting to consider how mindfulness may or may not be useful.

In most cases we do a practice together and work out any adaptations (e.g. for trauma, anxiety, a particular bodily challenge, cognitive difficulties, etc.), and sometimes a different route is taken (e.g. 1:1 mindfulness-based therapy, onward referral, a community-based course).

Ensuring people take the course at the right time for them is an important part of this, and sometimes there can be contact over several months while this is being ascertained. There can be tendency for people to want to start as soon as they are offered something as they are aware of NHS waiting lists. To address this, we have developed systems so that people can attend at a time it is appropriate for them, and courses offered at different times of day make that possible.

The initial meeting does several things, but not least, everyone will have met one of the therapists running the course and have a shared understanding of how they may be working with mindfulness. The box below gives a checklist of things that are considered from a notes review and/or discussion with the participant. However, it needs to be borne in mind that developing a relationship is important and that the therapist and participant need to 'meet' to understand more about each other and the programme; this rapport-building helps the course feel more comfortable and hopefully means the participant feels comfortable to get in touch. I then introduce myself and share something of my own practice and how the group was started. The point of the meeting is to find out more about the participant's situation and how mindfulness could help.

MINDFULNESS INITIAL MEETING

- Diagnosis/presenting physical health problem (ME/CFS, fibro-myalgia, Long Covid, chronic pain)
- Other health issues?
- Mental health diagnosis?
- Physical limitations
- Trauma
- Current mood, including suicide risk
- Other services involved now and in the past
- Social situation – housing/family/work, etc.
- Reason for referral (patient's perspective)
- Experience of mindfulness to date
- Experience of mindfulness in the session (do body and breath awareness practice, check for physical and emotional aversion and reactions indicating trauma)
- Any specific adaptations required? (physical, emotional, sensory, practice-related)
- Support during the course?
- Timing of course for both the sessions and the home practice
- Anything else.

From this, we consider the specific intentions of the course, and a note of these is made in the group spreadsheet, so we check in with the individual participant's intentions and formulate a goal for treatment (Bisseling et al. 2019). Each individual has their own reasons for starting the course, which may be:

- wants to work on acceptance
- would like to improve rest and manage wandering mind and also be in contact with people living with ME/CFS
- having done a mindfulness group before privately, is keen to revisit now they have Long Covid
- has anxiety, aware that this is a barrier, has been looking at regulation-type work and is keen to try a mindfulness approach
- has been doing meditation, finds somatic practices particularly helpful, is interested in the application of practices in day-to-day life
- would value the opportunity to establish a routine and to improve self-care.

Running the programme
Administrative support

This is an important factor in the smooth running of the programme. I have a full clinical caseload and other areas of responsibility (and am not the best at administration!). Support with making sure everyone is added to the list, then sent information and appointments, group dates, and so on, has been crucial and ensures there is a flow through the year of individual and group appointments. Having someone else to contact people who do not come or get in touch hopefully means they can be more honest about what their needs are, and we can find a way to help either with mindfulness or another approach.

The room or Zoom

Practical arrangements for running the group in a room included having enough space for people to lie down and for moving around and chairs of different sizes and shapes. Additionally, we had blocks for foot support and some yoga mats and bolsters, loads of pillows and blankets and some wooden meditation stools paid for by the hospital charity. We also had tea-making facilities and a contribution box so we could buy a range of teas. The rooms we have worked in have not always been the most pleasant and rarely quiet. The priority was that people felt comfortable and that as clinicians we could access the rooms with all the 'stuff' we needed.

In 2020, because of the pandemic, these arrangements became redundant and we had to learn how to run Zoom rooms. This has its own set of challenges:

both staff and participants having to learn new technology; having to adapt the programme to online delivery, including the use of slides; finding ways to interact with participants; not being able to see all participants; and, for example in movement sessions, uncertainty about what they were doing or any problems that arose. However, one upshot has been that the programme is now more accessible to those who cannot travel. There is still work to do for the more severely affected and disabled participants, but this is more possible with Zoom. As there is no need for travel, people can participate from bed, and we enable people to participate at their own pace; they can leave if they wish. The plan going forward is to have a mix of room and Zoom groups. We use the Zoom platform because of its ease of use, the breakout rooms and ease of access.

Follow-up

The end of the course is not the end of the programme. Everyone has an individual follow-up appointment about a month or so after the course has finished to consider how they are using mindfulness, and any particular changes, thoughts or reflections. This is also an opportunity to review self-management strategies and issues such as return to work where relevant.

Follow-on groups

Every month there are follow-on groups, which are now on Zoom and likely to remain so as the numbers are too large for our rooms, but this may be reviewed in the future. It is an opportunity to connect in with the practice and how this is supporting life going forward (see box). There is a general check-in, and normally a theme emerges for the practice and small group discussions. In the small groups, there is an opportunity to meet with four or five others in a separate online room to share what they wish. Often, there is a theme, such as reflecting on how their mindfulness practice is now; how they are resting; what they are noticing that supports their day-to-day life; or how they are managing setbacks. This builds on the work in the main course and is a chance to review where one is now. Sometimes, it is an opportunity to try other practices, and it was in these sessions that the adaptations to the group practices were developed.

FORMAT FOR FOLLOW-ON SESSIONS (ONE HOUR)

- 5–10 minutes: general check-in
- 20–30 minutes: practice
- 5–10 minutes: group inquiry

- 10–15 minutes: small group (optional and some people leave at this point)
- 5–10 minutes: feedback and final closing practice.

Follow-on group administration practicalities

We have no restriction on how many sessions people attend; there is a list of emails on a separate spreadsheet and people are emailed and invited to the session. They don't need to let us know they are coming, they can just come, and we record attendance in line with current confidentiality policy. Every two years or so we check if everyone still wants to be on the list and ask them to opt in. A surprising outcome was the number of people who emailed in saying they would never be able to come but would like to stay on the list because it reminded them to practise. With that in mind, sometimes links to other mindfulness information or a short reflection on the themes of the last session are added to the email.

We use the Zoom follow-up sessions and the email list to share information and also to gain feedback about the fatigue and pain service.

SUMMARY

- In order to run a full mindfulness course there needs to be flow of referral into the programme and time to meet everyone individually and ascertain their needs and goals for the session.
- While pre-pandemic, we ran entirely in-room sessions; since April 2020, we have been entirely online and have found this has increased access to the programme as more disabled people were able to attend with online adjustments.
- Following up in individual and group appointments enables carry-over of principles into daily life, and the monthly group follow-on sessions provide support and community.

Chapter 17

The Mindfulness Course

- Course adaptations
- Weekly session outlines and rationales

Before going into detail about the course, this quote from Saki Santorelli at the beginning of the mindfulness-based stress reduction (MBSR) curriculum guide is a helpful reminder of what we are doing:

Ultimately, and in a very palpable way, the 'curriculum' of MBSR is none other than your life and the lives of the people you'll share in and engage with week by week in the classroom. The suffering, the inconstancy, the lack of a solid, concrete 'self' – the wish for relief of suffering and the longing for well-being that you carry within you, and all the people you'll ever work with carry within them – is the curriculum, the vital life of MBSR. (Santorelli et al. 2017)

Overview of sessions and adaptations

All sessions became two hours long at a fortnightly frequency; although there was a case for shorter and longer sessions, this was the almost unanimous preference. Having the sessions fortnightly meant that people could manage their time and come to the group but also manage the rest of their lives. For some, one outing a week was all they could manage, and attendance was affected in the more frequent sessions. The cognitive challenges were referred to, and the longer gaps between sessions meant that people found they had time to become accustomed to the practices. The groups look very similar to a mindfulness-based cognitive therapy (MBCT) programme with changes in nuance and detail. They now all run over 16 weeks. In the timetables given below, timings are given for afternoon sessions, which start at 1:30pm; morning sessions start at 10:30am and follow the same schedule.

Sessions 1 and 3 are broadly unchanged from an MBCT programme. Practices are adapted in those sessions for the needs of the group.

Session 2 has been changed to 'Resourcing ourselves' and looks at grounding and regulation skills rather than the 'walking down the street' exercise. We felt this built on dealing with barriers, and developed skills and understanding that were emerging from the body scan to regulate up and down, and prepared participants for dealing with staying present and managing difficulty. Noticing the anatomy of an emotion (Bartley 2011) – thoughts, feelings, sensations and behaviours – is explicitly drawn out in the pleasant/unpleasant events discussions.

Session 4, 'Staying present', includes using the three emotional regulation systems from compassion-focused therapy (Gilbert 2020; Gilbert and Choden 2013) as an overlay to describe our responses. This map works with the boom-and-bust experience of people doing the course, and this session explores the Drive and Soothing elements further.

Session 5, 'Being with difficulty', explores the protective system and the stress reaction emphasizing turning towards and being with (as in Session 5 of MBCT/MBSR).

Session 6 considers how thoughts may affect these systems within the boom-and-bust cycle.

Session 7 looks at nurturing/depleting activity and the importance of a balanced Drive system and relapse management using the 'pit' diagram from the fatigue and pain-management programmes.

Following the seven weekly sessions, there are individual sessions and regular group follow-ups.

The orientation of the course is outlined in Table 17.1.

Table 17.1 Orientation

Activity suggestion	Rationale/notes
One hour at the most; other sessions will be two hours with a ten-minute break.	Opportunity to meet everyone else who may be doing the course; part of opting in.
Technical – being comfortable with Zoom – muting self and turning video on and off; chat function.	To learn how to Zoom without pressure of being in the group.
PowerPoint presentation of information about the course, how to make the most of it.	Overview of skills that will be taught and the approach. Opportunity for participants to check this is what they would like/want.
Ground rules and group agreements. PowerPoint and discussion.	Safety and comfort within the group, including the way breakout rooms will be managed.
Short practice and discussion.	An experience of a mindfulness practice in this setting and the discussion afterwards.
Breakout rooms for seven minutes (introduce each other, possibly share something you are happy to share, maybe why you want to do the course?).	To practise and experience breakout rooms that are used throughout the course and meet others in small group.

Reconvene as whole group, any reflections from the group, etc.	Bringing group back together, opportunity to hear from others, also modelling how course will be run.
Technical – accessing recordings, handouts, etc. Choices – can have handouts printed, etc.	Part of expectation of the course is to do the practices throughout the week. We try to be as accommodating as we can about resources.
Support during the course – can access via email to arrange a 1:1 appointment. Will be explicitly offered throughout the group and at the end.	Ensure people feel they can get help if they don't 'get it'. There are different ways to access the practices and approach so they are useful for each person – aim of group is for people to end up with their own way of using mindfulness-based practices.
Short practice and inquiry.	Models how the sessions will be run, another opportunity to experience the practice as a group.
People then email in to confirm their place, and a link to group sessions is sent.	Opting into the group; any questions/ challenges can be addressed rather than people dropping out from the service because they are uncomfortable with the approach or the medium.

Session 1: Theme – automatic pilot

This session is very much the standard MBCT/MBSR format. Adaptations will be within the practices and inquiry as outlined in previous chapters.

Time	Activity suggestion	Rationale/notes
1:30	Introductions to team; agreements/ ground rules review.	Welcome.
1:40	Short arrival practice, ending with inquiry about hopes for this course and what will support and help you.	A mindful way to start a course; individual intentions and needs listened for as well as whole group.
1:45	Hopes for the course (5 mins in threes and fours in breakout rooms). Give permission to not go into the breakout rooms, can stay in main room with facilitators. Feedback in main group. Don't ask everyone to contribute, can use chat as well as speaking. Remind people not to share anyone else's experience – share own thoughts, reflections. etc. Emphasize willingness to see what happens, holding hopes lightly.	To meet others and start to articulate hopes for course. Small group can help increase confidence at talking. Some evidence that being in breakout rooms of more than two is less stressful; also means if someone's broadband drops, there will hopefully be another person there. Choices in how to participate support the underlying themes and intention of the group – making wise choices. And to experience curious inquiry and non-judgement from clinicians. Also models working within current baselines.

cont.

Time	Activity suggestion	Rationale/notes
2:00	Raisin exercise – or any small item of food. Definition of mindfulness – what did we do with the raisin? Write up on a PowerPoint slide the process of how we experienced the raisin – one thing at a time, using senses, on purpose, curious, aware of judgement but non-judgementally, etc.	Capture experiences, sensations, thoughts, memories, etc., what it felt like, pleasant, relaxing, uncomfortable because I don't like raisins. An experiential definition of mindfulness, drawing this out from the group so the resulting slide is a definition that comes from the group. Can then refer to Kabat-Zinn's (2013) definition: 'Mindfulness is awareness that arises through paying attention, on purpose, in the present moment, non-judgementally.'
2:30	Break.	Possibly invite people to have a cup of tea mindfully.
2:40	Body scan and inquiry. Time on set up of posture: see notes on practice guidance.	Body scan is likely to be short but do go through the whole body so participants have an experience of this. Inquiry – broad inquiry into what was noticed, check for a variety of different experiences and also for commonalities – creating links across the group and validating a variety of experiences.
3:05	Volunteer's experience of the course and home practice.	Hearing previous participant experience and how they are currently using a mindfulness approach has been shown to be very helpful.
3:15	Home practice – planning and discussion.	If time, nice to do the planning in small groups. Identify barriers and reiterate the need to 'make it happen'; mindfulness is intentional and a Doing mind will often find reasons to not do it.
3:25	Finishing practice.	Closing the group, a moment to reflect on what has been experienced and to pause before going into the rest of the day.

Session 2: Resourcing ourselves – coming to the body

This session is similar to but different from MBCT and MBSR; the practices remain the same. We have found it helpful to focus on the body as a resource and the use of mindfulness in self-care. This also introduces the idea that awareness can be helpful, but also challenging, and that we can become aware not only of good things/bad things but what we can actively do to self-manage. The window of tolerance model is used to visually describe what is happening and how we manage using a sailing analogy.

Time	Activity suggestion	Rationale/notes
1:30	Arriving in the 'room', welcome, etc.	Welcome, setting the tone for the session, informal, friendly. Encouraging comfort.
1:40	Body scan and inquiry. (set up breakout rooms)	If possible, a different therapist leads the session for a different approach. Inquiry focusing on this practice, not the practice that has been done at home. If difficulties arise, exploring what happened and also focusing on what the person did to stay with it (i.e. highlighting existing resourcing strategies).
2:15	Home work discussion – ten minutes in small groups followed by a short plenary session (approximately five minutes).	Common issues that arise include finding the time to practise; wandering mind; falling asleep; finding pain difficult; finding the noises on the recording/the voice annoying; etc. The inquiry into this is an opportunity to experience non-judgemental curiosity, notice the nature of the mind and human experience and also become aware that others experience the same thing. This is an opportunity to explore the potential of mindfulness beyond a relaxation technique. See the arrows slide in the PowerPoint.
2:30	Break.	
2:40	Finding anchor points (breath, feet, movement, contact with the chair, etc.) – see practice guidance notes. Inquiry, encouraging investigation into what is grounding, anchoring. Investigating what someone did if they felt off-kilter.	In Session 2 this is often a breath-based practice. While it is important to give the experience of the breath, starting at the peripheries and using other senses can give people more options. Gently exploring the breath as movement in parts of the body – experiencing the breath as it is here and now rather than thinking about the breath.

cont.

Time	Activity suggestion	Rationale/notes
2:55	Window of tolerance and boom and bust (PowerPoint slide). Describe this as a group and also add in link to boom-and-bust cycle seen in fatigue and pain conditions. Introducing idea we can take action; mindfulness is not just about noticing, we can notice and make changes, regulate self and take care of self, including asking for help. Link back to anchoring practice and question 'How can I take care of myself?'.	Spend time on describing central section – life's ups and downs and how they are managed. The choppy waters (hyper and hypo) elements can happen and mindfulness gives the opportunity to be aware and take action, metaphor of improving our sailing skills in challenging waters (not about avoiding or even 'coping' all the time – acknowledging what is happening and taking care of self rather than self-improvement).
3:15	Home work discussion – the body scan, anchoring, pleasant events.	Appreciating when we are coping, pleasant events, good times – see Rick Hanson's work on placing our attention on positive, nurturing and nourishing experiences and actively taking in positive moments (Hanson et al. 2021).
3:25	Anchoring plus poem. The focus on the experience of 'the pleasant event' and how that feels starts to show how awareness of the surroundings and where we are can lead to a feeling of connection, nourishment and calming. Sometimes we read this passage written by Anaïs Nin (1975) that links presence with nature and the feeling that can arise: You exist by your smile and your presence. You exist for your joys and your relaxations. You exist in nature. You are part of the glittering sea, and part of the luscious, well-nourished plants, you are wedded to the sun, you are immersed in timelessness, only the present counts, and from the present you extract all the essences which can nourish the senses, and so the nerves are still, the mind is quiet.	Chance to practise anchoring again, and also poem to remind of paying attention to things that are OK.

Session 3: How do I feel when I move?

There is a lot of practice this week; the breath practice is developed but is explored with other anchors (other bodily sensations or sound or vision), giving some choice. The breath is useful in mindfulness as it directly connects us to now and can also give some indication of how we are. We can also control it and use it to support uncomfortable sensations (e.g. breathing out or into an area of pain).

Movement is introduced; the inquiry into what happens is often rich here and can show up how we approach all activity and movement. Noticing habits and patterns of, for example, always pushing, 'doing my best' or 'doing what I'm told' can be explored.

This session can often be emotionally charged as people connect with loss for their physical function. Being with this and seeing what is here now in a tangible way can support this. Movement can also tap into what helps – for example, changing posture can affect mood (and vice versa).

Time	Activity suggestion	Rationale/notes
1:30	Arrival, welcome, etc.	
1:35	Breath awareness practice (start with anchors so there is somewhere to come back to) and inquiry.	See last week's session plus practice guidance notes.
2:00	Home practice breakout rooms, then convene with whole group.	Ongoing opportunity for participants to meet each other, share what they are learning, etc. Whole-group discussion, continue to look at what supports home practice.
2:20	Break.	Ponder pleasant events.
2:30	Pleasant events: what do we notice? Bring to mind a pleasant experience right now (could be one you have written about or a new one). How do you know it is pleasant? What do you feel in your body? Emotions? Thoughts? Drawing out thoughts, feelings, emotions – the 'anatomy' of an emotion. Noticing transient and changing nature of experience and the joy of savouring the pleasant. Metaphor of cake or vase of flowers?	Table on PowerPoint to work through to look at an emotion, focus on bodily experience – how do we know we feel calm, happy, etc., what does it feel like? Draw out noticing small things, and also the fact the brain will tend to skim over 'OK' things, particularly if there is stress or pain as we are wired to react to unpleasant events.
2:45	Breathing space/anchoring pause: show PowerPoint slide. And do a short practice.	See practice guidance notes. Build on previous exercise by finding something that is OK right now, and using this to anchor. Part of the whole course theme of finding internal resources is preparation for later work on turning towards the more challenging aspects of experience. This is also building implicit compassion.

cont.

Time	Activity suggestion	Rationale/notes
2:55	Inquiry into what is noted, feelings, thoughts and sensations. What's familiar, what is new? How does it feel when I move? Led movement practice, possibly using the stretches used in pain- and fatigue-management programmes.	Continuing to resource ourselves through the body. Can be an opportunity to notice habits of pushing, following instructions... An opportunity to find individual edges. Finding a restful way to move and an active way to rest?
3:20	Home practice. Movement playing with edges. Noticing our response to unpleasant experience.	A range of options for movement practice is given – video link on the website, audio recording, images in the handout or a short walk. Having a range allows people to find their own movement practice according to how they are now. Some of the movements they will have met before in the physiotherapy sessions. Encouraging people to experiment and notice when they have pushed it or avoided. The 'unpleasant events' diary is a follow-on from the 'pleasant events' this week, and people are directed to notice small annoyances or vexations and the thoughts, sensations and emotions that arise.
3:25	Closing practice. Poem by Rumi: This fragment of Rumi's writing is often used in the session to reflect the hand movements we start with in the movement section of this session. Focus on the opening and closing and the detailed awareness we can cultivate in seemingly small movements that may seem like nothing, yet the allusion to wings and flight suggest freedom in movement. Your hand opens and closes, opens and closes. If it were always a fist or always stretched open, you would be paralysed. Your deepest presence is in every small contracting and expanding, the two as beautifully balanced and coordinated as birds' wings.	

Session 4: Staying present

Being with all of our experiences, including reactions to annoyances. This session starts to map our reactions and to introduce the idea that this may not be personal but is part of the human experience. The three-systems model described in compassion-focused therapy (Gilbert 2020; Gilbert and Choden 2013) provides a framework for noticing which system we are in and how this may affect what we think and do. It also gives us the opportunity to nurture some systems that may have been neglected, the Soothing system in particular. This system can link to the Being mode of mind and is not a place we often automatically find ourselves in; we often have to take ourselves there intentionally, and if we do find ourselves there, spend time appreciating and savouring it.

Time	Activity suggestion	Rationale/notes
1:30	Arrival, welcome, etc.	As per previous weeks.
1:35	Movement practice and inquiry.	Building from last week's session, also conversation about movement as personal practice in the previous fortnight.
2:10	Home practice discussion in breakout rooms, then convene with whole group.	Longer in breakout rooms as people are now getting to know each other and have more awareness of how the course is structured and what mindfulness is.
2:30	Break.	
2:40	Unpleasant events – mapping the experience. Bring to mind a small annoyance/irritation or notice something that is irritating right now; as you notice it, be curious about how you feel, the emotion, how that feels physically, what thoughts you have… Ask people to share their experience, focusing on thoughts, feelings and sensations and what they want to do (try to move away from the story of the event or, if they are caught up in it, reflect back the emotion, maybe what you are noticing yourself as you hear the story). Capture this on prepared PowerPoint slide or whiteboard. Conversation about how we respond to difficulty. What happens when we notice our reaction?	This exercise disrupts the idea that it is the annoyance that leads us to feel this way and instead focuses on the reactions we have, how they can vary and the physical and mental components to that reaction. It also introduces the idea that 'turning towards' difficulty doesn't make it worse, it can mean we deal with and respond to both the situation and our reaction and also watch it pass and change. Hearing how others react can help depersonalize and reduce self-blame.

cont.

Time	Activity suggestion	Rationale/notes
2:50	Anchoring practice. Awareness practice – body, breath, sounds, thoughts.	This practice serves as a break in the session and also as a way of responding to reactions by being aware of our reactions and using anchors to steady.
2:55	Emotional systems. Knowing which system we are in (draw out and discuss). Discuss the systems, then explore the Soothing system to enable approach mode – responding not reacting – practices and activity. Discuss what we consciously do to soothe ourselves – perhaps it's just noticing and being gentle, maybe something else – identify attitudes and things we can do to encourage this consciously (name in the chat something you can try).	Compassion-focused therapy circles model helpful to nuance further our observation of our reactions and also locate reactions as part of how we have evolved and function as a species; it's not our fault. Starting to identify how we have ways of soothing ourselves historically and also what is being learnt through the course.
3:15	Pause – anchoring.	Again a break, but actively accessing Soothing system and Being mode of mind.
3:20	Home practice planning – movement alternating with sitting, pausing, peace with gravity. Poem – possibly 'Gravity' by Rilke.	

Session 5: Being with difficulty

This session builds on the theme of the last session, being present with pleasant, unpleasant and neutral events, and takes it further by examining what happens when we withdraw, contract and resist difficulty, particularly the difficulty that will not go away. This has particular relevance for those living with challenging symptoms and the restrictions their health may place upon them. The metaphor of the second arrow is key to this session. It is important that people maintain autonomy and go at their own pace, hence the invitation to turn towards the smaller challenges and also to work with challenging thoughts by noticing the feeling tone within the body; for example, I may have a repetitive worry in my mind – rather than working with that directly, I can notice where I am holding tension (that may well be increasing other symptoms) and take care of myself by tending to that.

By interrupting the extra layers of stress, there is an opportunity to settle, which then enables the more creative aspects of the mind that can see other options to come 'online' as we are no longer solely in the protective fight/flight mode.

Sometimes, the 'turning towards' is very tentative, and it is at this point when 'taking a peek' at where the challenge is located it is possible to find a way to take care of oneself right there. By going too fast too soon, aversion can arise, and that can lead to additional stress and distress, upsetting things further.

This approach is supported by the work we have done so far on grounding, settling and soothing, so there is already an experience that attention can be placed in different areas and there can be moment-by-moment changes. The curious approach we have been encouraging is key here and the metaphor of a botanist vs. weed control when coming across an unfamiliar plant can be helpful. Additionally, we invite people to check out how they have coped, what they already do, emphasizing existing skills and resources in the inquiry. We note that working with difficulty is the transformative element of the course, not just calming down; being with difficulty can change our relationship to challenge.

Time	Activity suggestion	Rationale/notes
1:35	Arrival, perhaps with some movement practice.	
1:40	Finger trap experience (short online video shared). Discuss what it feels like to be stuck and what our instinct is – to pull away, what does that feel like? Direct attention to centre of the body – often, there is a clenching, breath-holding experience.	An explanation of the concept of what happens when we move towards rather than pull away when we are stuck. Probably better if we have finger traps, but the video clip demonstrates it well, and in the discussion someone usually knows you have to move towards and make space in order to get out of the trap.
1:55	Being-with-difficulty practice – body, breath, sounds, difficulty and then poem before inquiry. Poem: The Guest House. After inquiry and poem check people are OK and invite movement, grounding, shaking out if necessary	Spending time settling and an awareness of how the mind can place attention where we choose. Then choosing a current (in-the-moment) challenge rather than bringing a difficulty to mind – e.g. temperature, stiffness, worrying thought – and placing attention on the felt experience of that problem. If there is no current difficulty (rare!!) then offer the opportunity to enjoy this and savour the moment. Inquiry can help people explore where they felt it, what happened, perhaps how it changed; and if necessary, they can move on to how they resourced themselves through that moment. It is important to stay with what happened and not problem-solve.

cont.

Time	Activity suggestion	Rationale/notes
2:20	Break.	Perhaps reflect on the half-way review questions.
2:30	Home practice review in breakout rooms in threes. Half-way review – What am I noticing? How can I make the most of the rest of this course? Feed back to the whole group.	In whole-group, feedback can be helpful to place emphasis on those who have established patterns of regular practice and how they have done that and also emphasize the research evidence and advantage of longer practices. The longer practices offer more time, intentionally placing attention and practising compassion to self, and there is also more likely to be difficulty to deal with when doing a longer practice. How we deal with difficulty is perhaps the whole point of what we are doing.
2:50	Sea of reactions, pause and reflect on reactions to difficulty – What do we do? Each person either calls out or adds to the chat, facilitator collates information on whiteboard.	See MBCT for cancer (Bartley 2011). Gathering up our reactions, some may be more wholesome than others but noticing that we are trying to make ourselves feel better and often the difficulty cannot be changed. Note that mindfulness practices can be used in this way too (see 'spiritual bypassing' for more on this, helpful if facilitators are aware of when they do this both for themselves and also for the participants – we all want less pain and suffering for ourselves and others). Awareness and response rather than reaction can be transformative. Sometimes all we can do is be aware of what is going on.
3:00	Exercise in pairs – How do I know I'm stressed or in Threat mode? – staying with bodily experiences.	Choose a reaction and notice where you feel it in your body, possibly working with the diagram you've either drawn or the one that's in the workbook.
3:10	Feed back to the whole group, collect on a diagram drawn on the whiteboard.	Staying with the bodily reaction, can refer to the three-circles model – the Threat/protective mode. This reinforces that it is not 'pathological' or wrong to feel these symptoms, rather it is understandable, and the protection system is doing what it does best but perhaps other systems are needed, particularly the Soothing system.

| 3:20 | Pause/breathing space. | A break in the session but also to emphasize the 'what's up for me' inquiry that the pause can bring and the choices we can make when we notice and gently turn towards our current experience. |
| 3:25 | Home practice planning – sitting, challenging times practice if you wish, try some days without guidance. | Mention the insight timer app. Offer 1:1 support if needed. |

Session 6: Thoughts aren't facts

This session is very much the same as Session 6 in MBCT for depression but with an emphasis on thoughts that are prevalent in fatigue and pain conditions. The image of the boom-and-bust cycle is used to elicit the different thoughts and their consequences. The group is powerful in reinforcing the reality that often people living with these health conditions have very similar thoughts and experiences and that difficult thoughts as well as the boom-and-bust cycle are part of living with the health condition. This common experience can generate more self-compassion and a feeling of being understood by others. Giving time to capture the array of thoughts is important to cultivate this. Please see chapter 13 for more detail.

Time	Activity suggestion	Rationale/notes
1:30	Arrival with short movement practice. PowerPoint with images of how thoughts can be observed. Awareness practice – body, breath, sounds, thoughts – plus inquiry.	MBCT practice of observing thoughts. Emphasize that the practice doesn't have to be done while seated. Inquiry in depth with a few and widen the conversation to encompass possible array of experience – acknowledge sometimes we are aware of no thoughts. Transient and fleeting changeable nature of thoughts and challenge to locate them.

cont.

Time	Activity suggestion	Rationale/notes
2:05 (approx.)	Common thoughts in fatiguing syndromes, handout on screen – discussion (see chapter 13).	Pause on the list of thoughts, ask people to identify if they know any of these thoughts that have been elicited in interviews – emphasize the normality and commonality of these thoughts for people in this situation to the extent that they could be considered one of the symptoms. Depersonalizing, reducing self-blame for thoughts.
After the discussion	Pause.	As a break in the session and also building on the 'what's up for me?' and 'how can I take care of myself?' inquiring use of this short practice.
2:15	Role of thoughts in boom and bust – what drives them and what is the impact? PowerPoint with boom and bust drawn on – annotate with the group.	More detail into the thoughts, chance to discuss what thoughts are experienced by the group. (See chapter 13.)
2:30	Break.	
2:45	Small groups reflect on thoughts in boom and bust– What are the choice points? How can we work with these thoughts?	Encourage conversations to focus on how thoughts can be worked with using mindful awareness rather than the cognitive therapy process of challenging the veracity or helpfulness of thoughts.
2:50	Whole-group review of role of thoughts.	Continue with PowerPoint – emphasize choice points and supportive attitudes.
3:10	Home practice review and planning.	
3:25	Poem: 'An Autobiography in Five Chapters' by Portia Nelson and closing practice.	This poem emphasizes the compassionate point that we do not need to get it right each time. This is work in progress. Particularly, the boom-and-bust and cyclical nature of symptoms is likely to continue, but we can perhaps find options to work constructively with it rather than exacerbate and spiral down.

Session 7: Taking care of myself – integrating mindfulness into daily life

We have been asking 'How can I take care of myself?' throughout the course. It is perhaps an obvious question, but often people are more likely to ask of themselves 'How can I be better?' or 'How can I improve?'. This is the last session of this course but perhaps just the beginning of using mindfulness in a pragmatic way to support not only health but also the way of life and activities we want.

This is a full session as we are using concepts from both Sessions 7 and 8 in the MBCT/MBSR curriculum. It is important not to rush it; this plan seems to work, and giving pauses to reflect, speak, and so on, allows the theme to unfold. Individual sessions are offered at the end to explore further.

Time	Activity suggestion	Rationale/notes
1:30	Body scan and inquiry – draw out contrast from start of the course to the end.	Marking the end of the course by returning to the beginning, highlighting the process that there is nowhere to go and the attitudes of beginner's mind, curiosity into this current experience. Also an opportunity to reflect on how the practice has developed over the months.
2:00	Role of activity – hot-air balloon activity (drawn on a slide we add to during the session): please see chapter 14 for more details.	Based on nourishing and depleting activity, very similar to MBSR programme, with the acknowledgement that although some activities can be depleting in terms of fatigue, there is a benefit particularly in a baselined or little-and-often approach. Attitude to how we approach activity, drawing on the three compassion-focused therapy systems – we can make anything into a Drive/achieving activity. How do we keep it uplifting and enjoyable or allow it to give us enough of a sense of mastery?
2:15-ish	In small groups, looking at a typical day and how they can add to uplifting activity – reconvene as whole group.	Encourage people to support each other to look at how they can change activities from depleting to nourishing – facilitators can give personal examples.
2:30	Break.	

cont.

Time	Activity suggestion	Rationale/notes
2:40	Mindfulness at different times, when things are OK, when they start to get wobbly and when they are in a setback pit; use blank pit PowerPoint and populate together (see chapter 14).	This comes from the pain- and fatigue-management programmes and is an opportunity to explore strategies as well as mindfulness-based approaches. By actively planning for harder times, we are addressing the idea that recovery is always about improvement. Recovery (and life) is about how we navigate challenges, and while things can be hard, it is perhaps how we face our darkest times that we learn about ourselves and what is important to us in the best of times.
2:55	Home practice review – emphasis on what I will keep going and what support I will need.	Continuing on from above, what practice will we use now?
3:15	Group closing saying what they will take forward in discussion and in the chat.	
3:25	Poem.	Prelude to 'The Dance' by Oriah Mountain Dreamer. Interestingly, the author has chronic fatigue syndrome.

Chapter 18

Living with Fatigue

FROM DOING TO BEING

by Rhonda Knight

Rhonda Knight is a retired adult nursing lecturer living with ME/CFS, who attended the mindfulness course after doing a self-management programme. She has since become a patient volunteer and supports the course participants with her lived experience. Over the years, she has played a key role in developing the programme, and her reflections from her experience have informed how we work. Rhonda is also involved in patient audit and is a patient representative trustee and board member of the British Association of Clinicians in ME/CFS.

She writes: 'It took years for me to be diagnosed with ME/CFS and to get some help, but now my life has totally changed for the better and I am really enjoying life. Since retiring from lecturing in 2014, I still do some casual work playing the role of the patient for clinical learning experiences and exams. I really enjoy the contact with the students, as well as the voluntary work I do with North Bristol Trust as a patient facilitator in the mindfulness programme, plus being involved in research, audits, and whenever the input of patients is needed to inform policy and/or clinical practice. The following is my experience of ME/CFS and mindfulness.'

Diagnosis and living with ME/CFS

I had been feeling absolutely exhausted for several years. I had grown used to a certain level of fatigue following a bout of pleurisy when I was a teenager, and I had had frequent long periods off work with the diagnosis of depression. That never really felt quite right, and others seemed to have a different experience to me. The fatigue was accompanied by significant pain that moved around my body and repeated sore throats together with a loss of voice. I also realized that

I was having trouble with my memory, and my ability to prioritize tasks and make decisions was compromised. My reading, comprehension and writing skills were significantly affected. I had gone through a couple of years of hell, thinking I was either 'lazy', 'useless' or a 'failure', then convinced I was getting either dementia or multiple sclerosis (because of repeated falls) or that, yet again, I was depressed. I tried desperately to hide my inadequacies, particularly at work, which only increased my stress levels and feeling of exhaustion and pain.

In 2012, after a holiday where I was tired beyond belief, I eventually went to my GP. After many tests, I was referred to the ME/CFS clinic, where I was finally given the diagnosis of ME/CFS and fibromyalgia in January 2013.

Self-management programme

I found the initial information courses at the hospital really enlightening, realizing that lying on the sofa and snoozing all day was not helpful. I learnt how to make action plans with goals that were realistic, how to prioritize what I did and make changes in my life, such as shopping online, doing the ironing in small batches and setting a time limit on how long I would spend gardening. I found tremendous support and comfort from a cohort of patients that I met living with ME/CFS, and whose experience of living with such a condition resonated with my own experience. At last, I was able to work with a diagnosis that made sense of the cluster of symptoms that I often had.

My introduction to mindfulness

I first heard of mindfulness when I was a lecturer in Adult Nursing at the local university. Gilbert's (2010) book *The Compassionate Mind* was selected for a module's reading list, and, while dutifully reading it, I thought: how could being compassionate improve my well-being? If anything, my experience of being compassionate had led me to feel worn-out and fatigued, both mentally and physically.

The hardest part was 'teaching'/facilitating the students' compassionate learning experience. How could I teach it, when I struggled so much to be compassionate, not only towards my past patients, but also to my current students and colleagues, and especially to myself? I decided my mental health colleagues were 'fluffy, tree-hugging softies', and that I just didn't understand where they were coming from. It did not fit in with my biomedical background, and, at the time, I did not think it was relevant or have the necessary energy or time to research it.

I was invited to a mindfulness programme that was being developed within the ME/CFS service. I didn't really understand what I was committing myself to, but being the good student, I kept a reflective log and here are my thoughts as I went through the programme.

Reflections on the weekly sessions
Week 1: Automatic pilot

I was excited about attending the first session as 'mindfulness' must be something that could help me to live with my long-term condition, otherwise why would it be offered by the ME/CFS clinic? I was sceptical about any potential effectiveness of mindfulness though, but references to relevant research about how mindfulness could change brain activity for the better captured my attention. I don't mind admitting that after the session, I searched online for each reference, just to make sure that the 'wool wasn't being pulled over my eyes'! I wanted to *do* mindfulness to enable me to cope with the symptoms that limited my daily life, especially the poor concentration, inability to focus and disabling lack of attention.

The first session entitled 'The Automatic Pilot' was an interesting place to start my mindfulness journey. With the raisin exercise, I found it fascinating to have a close encounter with this particular raisin, using my senses to really get to know this piece of dried fruit. There was a myriad of colours ranging from red to deep purple and black, and at some angles, there was even a rainbow effect, probably from the waxy coating that develops during the dehydration process. The texture was rough and dimpled, yet it felt squishy and soft when squeezed between my fingers and left an unpleasant sticky mess. When invited, I popped it into my mouth and resisted the urge to give it a couple of chews and immediately swallow it. Just one bite released an overwhelming taste of sweetness, something that I had never experienced before, as usually I bolt down any food before being interrupted, probably an old habit from my nursing days. I did savour that sweet taste of this previously unseen raisin. I did not realize at the time, or even in the discussion that followed this exercise, that this close encounter with a raisin was an example of being mindful, being present in the here and now, and that I was using all my senses to experience that raisin. On reflection, I was aware of being very judgemental of the exercise – what a silly idea to have a sticky raisin to examine – I was too shy to excuse myself and go and wash my hands!

I was totally out of touch with the physical experience of my body and how and where I experienced emotions, such as fear, anger, joy, happiness or contentment. I did not even recognize the physical sensations of hunger or thirst. Where did I feel those emotions in my body? My curiosity was aroused when doing a guided body scan for the first time and realizing that I was unaware of what the sensations that I was feeling meant. There were parts of my body I could not feel, and I was fighting an overwhelming urge to not fall asleep. 'Good' students don't fall asleep in class!

In my desperation to find something that might help to live with such debilitating symptoms, I made a commitment to *do* the home practice regularly. I didn't understand why so much dedicated practice was necessary, or what the intended learning outcome might be, but I did know that when feeling stressed or under pressure, I am very good at procrastinating and find it difficult to be self-disciplined, especially when I don't understand the potential benefits. It was fortunate that I was not working at the time, as I would not have been able to devote the time to the home practice.

I settled down the day after the first session to do the 45-minute guided body scan, lying on a yoga mat and covering myself with a blanket, head supported by a pillow and arms resting by my side, palms upwards, just like it was suggested in the CD. What a nightmare. I either fell asleep, went into a daydream, was racked by familiar and excruciating pain, or else argued with the content of the guided commentary. In those days, my thinking was 'all or nothing' and I became really irritated by the 'fluffy nonsense' that I was repeatedly hearing. Breathe through my toes? Breathe out through my head? 'Get a grip, lungs are used for breathing!' Heads are for thinking; toes are for maintaining balance when walking...this was hard work!

As I was not able to *do* what was asked of me, maybe I was failing at *doing* mindfulness, even before I have started. As I continued with my daily home practice, I found that I could pretend to breathe in through my toes, but breathing out through my head was impossible. Pretending was the only strategy that I could think of in order to *do* this practice 'properly', but where was all this breath going? Was it trapped inside of me? Were the parts of my body that I couldn't feel – my toes, top of my feet, my kneecaps – missing? Slowly, I did become aware of tingling/burning sensations in my toes, legs and fingers, a shooting pain at the top of my right shin, twitching arms, transient itches, rumbling stomach – was that hunger or just my normal digestive processes? One noticeable observation was how thirsty I was after each body scan and I needed to down a glass or two of water, something I normally rarely drank, after each practice.

Often, I found that I slept until the final bell, when I woke with a start, was aware of my heart thumping, and not knowing where I was, the time of the day, what I was supposed to be doing or how long had I been asleep and with an overwhelming sense of tiredness. Maybe I'm not *doing* this right. A great internal battle raged, but still I clung on to the hope that by just *doing* the practice, I would make sense of it during the later stages of the programme, though I did wonder if I would ever master mindfulness. One of my personal attributes is my inherent sense of honesty, so I knew that I would not be able to fake any expected change due to mindfulness, either to myself or to others.

The practice that I enjoyed the most was being aware of routine activities – going for my usual daily walk, sitting in a different chair, cleaning my teeth, watching the kettle boil and making my coffee. Without realizing it at the time, I was beginning to be mindful and was astounded at the range of sights, smells and tastes that I had never noticed before when carrying out these very mundane activities. I had been missing out on so much; however, it would be a long time before I was able to start to recognize feelings, emotions and bodily sensations, and this is something that I am still exploring in my current mindfulness practice.

The second session loomed, and I was quite scared as I did not feel that I had been particularly successful at *doing* the body scan. It was a chore to do each day, and even though I had done it regularly, I resented the time spent doing it, feeling it was a waste of time. My toes were still refusing to breathe, and more often than not, I couldn't even feel them, which left me wondering if I did have any toes attached to my feet! This mindfulness practice wasn't making much of a difference to my symptoms or my life...

Week 2: Resourcing ourselves

The theme of the second session was 'Resourcing ourselves', with the aim of becoming aware more often. What that actually meant, I had no idea, but after last week's focus on 'automatic pilot', I realized that I had an awful lot to learn, as my only modus operandi was in mindless activity! Still, I was not put off in my exploration of such an outlandish way of thinking. I have always approached professional learning opportunities with a sense of curiosity. Little did I realize that my natural sense of curiosity was a core attribute of mindfulness practice, and that this innate talent would be the crux of my exploration of mindfulness.

After the welcome, we participated in another guided body scan, and it felt good to be doing it with other people in the same room. To me, it was a godsend, as it gave me the space and time to collect myself and recover from the stress of getting ready and driving to a morning session. I must admit that I felt a sense of achievement as I managed to stay awake throughout the *whole* of the body scan.

I was fascinated by the inquiry after the body scan, as people were mentioning themes that were similar to my doubts and struggles, and I realized that my experience was not unusual. One particular fellow participant intrigued me, as they mentioned their awareness of pain during the scan, and how they could 'see' the shape and colour of the pain. This was beyond the realm of my previous thinking and experience as a nurse, who assessed pain from a medical model of practice, inquiring about the onset, characteristic and location of their pain. I never thought about assessing myself or viewing the pain that I experienced so visually. Listening to the other patients in the small group talking about their home practice was also helpful as I did not feel so alone in my daily commitment. Our sharing began the formation process of an incredibly supportive group that continued to meet independently for about 18 months after the programme finished.

I was curious about developing an awareness of my breath, as it seemed that it might be a possible tool to use in my mindfulness practice, knowing that one's breath is always there. I was intrigued to learn what the benefit might be when we were invited to 'treat it as a friend'. My concrete thinking quickly stepped into play again. How can something so automatic like breathing be seen as a friend? Maybe 'familiar' would describe it better for me. Well, it was a challenge that I was willing to accept, little knowing how this activity would lead to such a change in how I responded emotionally and physically to stressful situations.

This week centred on the 'window of tolerance' (Siegel 1999) and thinking what triggers led to a state of either hyper- or hypo-arousal. I struggled with taking on new learning as I was significantly affected cognitively at the time and had little ability to focus or pay attention. Having the handout for the session was helpful though, as I could think about it at home and was able to identify the signs of sailing out of my window of tolerance: feeling anxious and tearful, eating junk food instead of proper meals, spending too much time doing mindless puzzles, and isolating myself from others by ignoring texts and emails. I decided that I could ground myself by focusing on my breathing, by going for a short daily walk to be aware of the natural world, and listening to music that reminded me of my safe and wild haven, an island away from the mainland and the demands of everyday life.

After the second session, the idea that the practice of mindfulness is not a competition, not even with myself, began to crystallize, but I was still struggling with the concept of breathing into my toes, and even experimented with trying to push the air down from my abdomen to see if that would work. I still worried about doing the exercise properly. The notes in the handout did explain that the only discipline is regular and frequent practice, and I had already made that commitment, but it was so hard to accept that there was no guarantee of a rapid, positive outcome. I was so geared up to achieving specific outcome measures in my professional life, and it just seemed ridiculous that the more I tried to influence what mindfulness would do for me, the less successful I would be. During the week, I struggled to be gentle with myself when I fell asleep during the practice, and especially when I missed a couple of days of practice as I had a relapse, experiencing fatigue and pain.

Just before the next session, I was curious enough to experiment during the body scan. I didn't force my breath into my toes, but just tried to let the breath drift down. Paradoxically, by not trying too hard, the visualization of my breath was more vivid. I started to feel sensations in various parts of my body, sometimes when I was focusing on that part of the body; at other times, sensations such as throbbing, stabbing, tingling, pulsating, itchy, heat and coolness, prickling, pressure, twitching, aching, cramping and burning in different parts of my body intruded and diverted my attention. Maybe, even the sensation of hunger! I didn't realize that I could feel so much in my body! It was a huge learning curve for me to stop striving and to be aware of what was happening in the here and now, accepting things as they are, and to have the faith to Just *Do* the Practice!

Initially, I did the breath exercise for three minutes, then noticed that the handout suggested that we practised it for 10–15 minutes each day. Oh dear! Was my miserly three-minute practice going to deliver any results? I tried to do the exercise for the 'proper' length of time and was amazed, as I did it on a day when I was experiencing so much pain in the base of my neck and across the top of my shoulders, scoring about an 8 on a scale of 0 to 10, where 10 was the most severe pain ever experienced. I really tried to focus on the area in my body where the pain was, and 'breathe' into my pain. This was a 'fluffy' visualization, and I had always dismissed past practice of visualization as just thoughts that would never affect how I felt physically, and maybe unaware of unconscious body/mind dualism. Encouraged by the revealing disclosure of a fellow patient during the session, I thought I would try it.

> 'I visualized inflating the pain with air, so that it was light enough to drift away.'

I was amazed how much the pain had decreased in ten minutes, with my perceived pain now scoring about 4 in intensity and at a level that I could cope with to continue with my day. This was an amazing experience and breakthrough, and it was only Week 2 of the programme!

During the week, I used the breathing exercise when experiencing other uncomfortable physical events, such as hip pain and nausea, when I noticed the sensation of thirst, something I usually was not aware of, so promptly made a drink, which did relieve the nausea. I learnt that by practising the breath exercise, it could be used as an effective tool in controlling the pain that I was finding so troublesome and debilitating, especially as it never seemed to respond to regular analgesia. What remarkable progress in my practice of *doing* mindfulness!

The practice that I did enjoy was the routine activity/habit releaser, watching a kettle boil and noting what I was observing in the here and now. It was a revelation to my 'automatic pilot' person. Obviously, I could hear the kettle boiling, but I could also smell the water when it was near to boiling and feel the heat coming from the kettle. What I was hearing also changed, from the initial crackle as the element started to heat, then the low bubble and popping sound to the final rush of boiling, bubbling water. I had never stood still long enough before or used my senses to observe a kettle boiling. There was so much happening!

However, when I went for an autumnal walk, I did hear the swishing of my feet amongst the dry leaves and saw the different colours of the leaves, as well as nuts and berries strewn on the ground, but I was more concerned about my appalling inability to identify which leaf came from which tree, and how I needed to do some research and learn to name each type of leaf. I commented that I was 'using my senses as I was walking', but it was only my sight and hearing. I was not aware of any other senses, or emotional or physical experiences. I did not know what my body was experiencing or even how my body moved when walking.

This week we had paper home work to do where we were asked to keep a positive events diary, noting whether we were aware of the accompanying pleasant feelings at the time, and where in the body we experienced such feelings, and record our mood, emotions and thoughts. It was an exercise that I struggled to start doing. 'Everything is always awful in my life at the moment. Nothing ever nice happens to me! So why bother with this exercise?' However, I did start to notice really small and fleeting positive events, such as babies or toddlers smiling or waving to me when I went out and socialized.

> 'I am so fortunate to have so many babies in my life at the moment who accept me as I am!'

As the week progressed, I found my voice and was able to explain to friends how I was really struggling with this ME/CFS 'thing'. I was overwhelmed by the many positive responses of offers and delivery of cooked meals, treats and bunches of flowers.

Noting the accompanying thoughts, emotions and where I felt them in my body was a challenge for me. I was aware of the muscles in my face lifting into a smile and the frown disappearing from my forehead, and a sense of warmth and lightness spreading across my chest, but some thoughts and feelings arising from a pleasant event were not always pleasant. I felt very guilty when hot meals were offered, and fearing that I was putting people out, I found my body tensing up, wanting to disappear, and I avoided making eye contact. As a result, I didn't always recognize the positive event as it was happening, but later when completing the diary, I was able to see things from other people's perspective – like the friends who must have been worried about me and offered to take me out for a short drive to do some birdwatching. The realization dawned that it was their way of helping me, as they had no idea how fatigue and post-exertional malaise could affect someone, never having been ill in their own lives. Completing the table after the event and reflecting on the positive event was helpful, as I started to notice positive thoughts, that normally I was totally unaware of.

> 'What wonderful friends I have who are willing to help me when I feel so under the weather!'

I had been struggling with the fact that my family lived in Australia, and I lived alone here in the UK, and that sense of isolation was reinforced when other participants spoke of the help and support they received from partners and family. My main conclusion from completing the positive event diary was that I don't *have* to have family close to hand to be cared for when feeling unwell. That profound insight into my support network here in the UK helped me to feel not so scared and alone in my struggle to live with the symptoms of ME/CFS. Compared to the start of the week, my perspective on life was beginning to change…

Week 3: How do I feel when I move?

This session's theme was 'breathing and moving' and was something that I really did struggle with as I had not been doing any exercise because of the level of fatigue that I was experiencing. I thought that I had to rest, rest, rest and, to be quite honest, I was quite apprehensive about this session. How much would I be expected to do? 'Movement' meant 'exercise' to me, and the thought of even going for a short 20-minute walk was more than I could contemplate, something that really grieved me as I had loved long-distance and hill walking in the past.

We started by doing a breath awareness practice together, which we had been practising at home. I was starting to understand that this might be a helpful technique in my everyday life, and so was interested to see if I had been *doing* it 'right'. It also gave me the time to collect myself again after arriving.

With frequent practice at home, I became more aware of the breath entering my nostrils, the coolness of the air entering, and the triangular shape it made just inside my nose. I was also aware of the dry patch at the back of the roof of my mouth as the breath was travelling down to my lungs, something which I had never noticed before, and the strangely soothing rhythmic movement of my lungs, diaphragm, chest wall and abdomen with each inhalation and exhalation. There was something reassuring going on here, but I didn't really understand what or why at that time.

I now use the breath awareness to ground myself when I once used to burst into tears in an automatic response to some stressful or emotional situation, where the intensity of my response to the situation used to confuse me and surprise those who were unfortunate to witness my unexpected emotional outburst. I had worked out in the past that it was in response to feeling powerless, angry (often justified) and threatened (often unjustified!).

When reflecting on our positive events diary in the group, there were two phrases that were mentioned by other participants that resonated with me and helped me to focus more on bodily sensations in response to emotions:

'Joy in my heart'

That's where I feel the happy/joyful emotions in my body.

'Can draw on the pleasant experiences at other times'

This comment I found very encouraging and have learnt to use my memory bank of pleasant events to relive those moments, and so feel more positive when I ponder and remember those memories and the associated emotions and bodily sensations.

The exercise for the coming week was to look at unpleasant events, though we were strongly cautioned not to choose major catastrophes but instead focus on those mildly annoying events that happen every day. I found completing this diary easier as I was more aware when things were 'going wrong'! It turned out to be a week of dropping things, probably because I was tired, not concentrating on the task in hand and also not being aware of where my body was and what it was doing. As usual, my brain, busy worrying how I was going to do everything that needed to be done when feeling so exhausted, was disconnected from my body.

I realized that I frequently held my breath and felt my throat tighten and ache followed by letting out a deep, low growl – no wonder I often had a sore throat! I have learnt that the sensation of my throat tightening is a key signal to use some form of mindful practice to give me the space to decide how to respond to any unpleasant event.

What really hit me though was the harshness of my judgemental thoughts:

'I am so clumsy!'
'Why am I so useless?'
'Why do I always make a mess when I have just tidied up?'
'Everything is such a big effort!'
'Why do I even bother to try and do anything?'

No wonder my self-esteem and confidence were at such a low ebb when constantly hearing those messages. The accompanying emotions were also interesting – frustration, annoyance, impatience and anger with myself, leaving me feeling like a failure, deflated, fed up and exhausted. But I still was failing to identify where in my body these emotions manifested themselves. I didn't have a clue!

When sharing what we had learnt from this exercise, my overwhelming insight was that pleasant events do happen in my life, even when I think that the majority of my existence is complicated by an avalanche of unpleasant ones. Life is not as desperate as I thought it was.

The movement part of the session was not as scary or physically exhausting as I was fearing, as it started with gentle movement of hands, head, neck and shoulders whilst we were still seated, then an invitation extended for a gentle stroll around the room if we felt able to. It was interesting that we weren't being pressurized to participate or do anything beyond our capabilities. I was also intrigued that the physical activity was called movement, rather than exercise. Exercise was still something I avoided at all costs in my attempt to look after myself, but perhaps it was possible to move. During the walking experience, though, I could not identify what part of my body was moving or any bodily sensations. There was no awareness or sensation of moving. Nothing!

I have thought long and hard about this since, as I am still challenged by being aware of how my body experiences moving in the physical environment. I had learnt to ignore my body and experience of pain after sustaining a nasty ankle fracture on a walking holiday, which resulted in multiple operations and the residual pain of traumatic arthritis. Every step was a nightmare, even on crutches; so to cope, I must have totally blocked out the sensation of pain, and any other physical sensations. I also think that my time nursing on the wards did not help with my self-awareness, as I never had time to eat or go to the toilet. I had trained myself to ignore those sensations of hunger, thirst and the need to 'spend a penny'! I am still learning to be aware of my body and noticing the often ignored messages about my physical, emotional and mental well-being. I continued with some short walks and realized that I was becoming more aware of the surroundings, as I usually walked with my head down, watching where I was walking, so that I didn't fall again and sustain another fracture.

I also did the gentle movement exercises at home whilst sitting down, closing and opening my fist, moving my head, neck and shoulders, and I made a startling discovery about myself. I looked down at my hands and saw the imprints of my fingernails embedded into my palms...and it hurt! The difference between the 'hard' and 'soft' edges of movement had been explained to us in the session. I realized that I always extended myself to be the best, go the furthest and fastest, so always reaching for the 'hard edge' when moving. A family saying when a child was 'If a job's worth doing, do it properly!'. I am still learning not to push myself to the extremes, either physically or cognitively, and maybe reaching for the soft edge is good enough, and that's OK!

I was alternating the movement practice with the body scan each day and was surprised to find that I was beginning to look forward to *doing* the scan. It was becoming part of my daily activity, and I no longer saw it as a chore that I had to *do*, but as something enjoyable. How did I enjoy it? Where did I feel that joy? I still had no idea, but I was falling asleep later in the guided meditation as I was aware of exploring parts of my body, such as my trunk and arms, not visited before.

It was about this time in the programme that the reality of living with a long-term condition was beginning to set in. Thanks to the courses that I had done before the mindfulness programme, it was gradually dawning on me that ME/CFS was something I had to live with, and that as yet there was no cure for this unpredictable and variable condition which impacted on my daily life. I was experiencing grief in its rawest form – anger, rage, despair, frustration, regret and a sense of loss for the times when I could achieve what I wanted, despite the heaviness of fatigue disabling me at other times. What I had really lost was that sense of hope that this was just a temporary blip, but no, this was something that I would have to learn to live with and I was angry. It was emotionally exhausting, and I had lost my sense of identity as a senior lecturer in adult nursing, thanks to ME/CFS.

At the end of this session, a reading of an excerpt of a poem by Rumi, a 13th-century Persian poet, resonated with me. It felt so true! I *was* 'bravely working' through my grief to make sense of the practice of mindfulness, even though at this stage, I still could not see, feel or really understand the benefits of this mystical practice. Hearing my struggle being acknowledged in such a confident way was somehow encouraging. My determination was renewed to commit to regular home practice. My curiosity was piqued, wondering what could happen if I were to continue with this routine. Maybe, just maybe, one day I would see my 'joyful face'!

Week 4: Staying present

The fourth session really made me reflect on how I was rarely present to what was happening in the here and now. I remembered daydreaming and living in an imaginary world with imaginary people during my childhood and teenage years. What was that all about? What was I escaping from? All I know was that it was a safe place, and the thought of even trying to be present was frightening and filled me with fear and dread.

We arrived at the session to a movement practice, and again I found the inquiry process, as well as the sharing of the home practice, fascinating and instrumental in developing my own knowledge and understanding. Listening to other people's experience of the practice, so often different to mine, was thought-provoking, especially when they described awareness of their body with such vivid pictures and images. The sharing of common emotions and their experience of frequent intruding thoughts was reassuring to me, as I still believed them to be unwanted interferences in my efforts to practise mindfulness. I recall not being able to be aware of what my body was doing when I was moving and the resulting frustrations and annoyance with myself because I obviously was not *doing* the practice properly. I was failing, even though I was trying so hard!

In the session, I was invited to feel the seat that I was sitting on, and I protested vigorously that I felt nothing. As I am sitting writing this, I can now feel the pressure of the chair on my 'sitting bones' (ischial tuberosities), the softness of the cushion supporting my back, my spine upright with my head balanced on top and my wrists and hands balancing over the keyboard with my fingers darting in different directions. Accompanying all this is a feeling of achievement and thankfulness that I learnt to touch-type, making this activity so much easier. Now that is, for me, some considerable progress!

We were taught short pauses, from Session 2, and I practised the three-step breathing exercise regularly each day, each time I boiled the kettle. Then I purposely started to notice my reactions to difficulties and stress. New insights about how I reacted and coped with stress were starting to emerge. I was still struggling to recognize any feelings in my body, perhaps because thoughts and emotions often overwhelmed me. But the short three-minute practice focusing on my breath was rhythmic and became reassuring and I delighted in exploring how I could feel my breath in various parts of my body.

One day, I was suddenly startled by something, and I noticed that I had stopped breathing completely. I became aware of how my breathing was affected when feeling stressed. I began to wonder whether my breathing (or lack of it) was key to my continual anxiety and impending sense of doom. Being perpetually in that place was exhausting, but from the increasing awareness of my body, albeit in small increments, I knew something was happening – at last!!

It was a couple of weeks later that I realized that I was using the breathing space/anchoring pause effectively for the first time. I had workmen in the house, always a stressful situation at the best of times. A new fire was being installed in the space left by my old gas fire and back boiler. It turned out that the new fire that I had chosen did not fit the hole left in the wall. I was aware of my throat tightening and aching, a physical forerunner to my inevitable tears in response to the electrician's frustration, which I misinterpreted as anger. Also, I felt 'very stupid'. 'How could I be so careless?' I noticed my breath. I had stopped breathing, and whilst the process of breathing again only took a few seconds, I suddenly saw the word 'mindfulness' drift into my thoughts.

Suddenly, I heard myself asking if anyone wanted a cup of tea, and so the electrician sat on the sofa drinking his tea, staring glumly at the dark, dusty space in my wall. When he had finished, he started to enlarge the hole and the new fireplace was eventually in place. The situation soon blew over. It was the first time in my life that I was aware of making a choice, rather than automatically bursting into tears. I had given myself a moment to ground myself and to choose a more appropriate action in response to what had happened. I was also aware of saying to myself, 'What do I need to do now to take care of myself?', words so often heard in the guided meditation sessions. By offering to make a cup of tea – a real 'nurse' activity which soothed both myself and others – I realized that by responding to upsetting events more calmly I was not wasting needless energy. This was a big breakthrough in my mindfulness journey.

In this session, the topic of the three emotional systems of Drive, Threat and Soothing was interesting to explore and widened my horizons to stay present and react to stressful situations in a more mindful way, rather than on automatic pilot. I always responded to events in an impulsive way, and in fact I believed that this was me and that it was impossible to *choose* how to react to an event. I was never aware of that split-second moment when a choice was possible. Realizing that I was usually operating from the driven system, needing to achieve a goal that was often impossible, or retreating from the world to protect myself from perceived threats that usually never materialized, was a wakeup call. I was aware of things that soothed me, walking, birdwatching, playing the piano, singing, watercolour painting, knitting and other crafts, but was always too busy to take them up. I had so many self-imposed deadlines that I had to meet.

The following week at home, I took up colouring, as I had found a mindfulness colouring book. I had always enjoyed this mindless activity when younger and had a beautiful set of coloured pencils. I realized that when I did it, I lost all track of time and my busy mind calmed down. It was a *mindful* activity, not a mindless one. I was surprised and still continue to make time for these activities, knowing that they are so important in helping me transition to a soothing emotional system.

The home practice for this week was alternating movement practice with a sitting meditation. Up until now, I had always done the body scan lying down on a yoga mat. I had briefly tried a meditation stool in a session and thought that using one might help my posture during the sitting meditation, as a chair was too uncomfortable. When using the stool, I found that I was able to stay awake for longer, though I did make sure that I was facing the sofa so there was something soft to fall on in case I did drop off to sleep. It was strange being in an upright posture, but at the same time I noted that I felt 'supported and held' by the stool. I felt that I was graduating to the next stage of mindfulness practice.

As I was doing the sitting meditation, still guided by the CD, I heard for the first time the words in the dialogue, 'being...human...whole', probably because I had not fallen asleep by this stage. The meaning of these words had not registered with me before. 'Whole?' I never thought of myself as being whole but broken and a non-achiever. The possibility arose that I could 'be whole', despite living with long-term conditions – post thyroidectomy, ME/CFS and impaired mobility due to an old, fractured ankle. That was something that I had never considered. I always tried to ignore my limitations, working through the pain, exhaustion, fatigue and cognitive fog. As a result, I had not been 'true to myself'. My concept of self was being severely challenged by this programme, with the possible outcome of self-acceptance, a new and very fragile thought.

During the meditations, I was starting to realize how busy my mind was, continually thinking ahead, planning and prioritizing what I had to do next – jobs that needed doing – but I was failing to plan any enjoyable activities. I didn't have time for that, and anyhow, did I really deserve it? Oh, how critical and harsh I was on myself!

I also realized that it didn't matter if I fell asleep during a body scan exercise. What was important was that I was aware that I had woken up from the nap, refocused on my breathing and continued with the meditation. The awareness of movement and its practice was still challenging, probably because I was attempting to do a yoga-type practice that was really beyond my physical capabilities at that time, but, as always, I had to stretch myself to prove that I could 'reach for the stars' and meet any challenge, no matter how ambitious and unrealistic the practice was in the light of the current limitations of my body. I am never going to be one to shy from a challenge.

However, I was beginning to gain some insight into what mindfulness might mean. It was not about doing exercises perfectly and it definitely was *not* a competition with either myself or anyone else. Perhaps mindfulness was more about being aware of what is happening in the here and now, not judging what I was experiencing or how effectively I was doing it, but allowing myself to just *be*, instead of always being on the go, trying to achieve some goal, which so often was unrealistic and affected my self-esteem and mental well-being so much.

The practice of 'making peace with gravity' by flopping down on the sofa whenever I sat down during the day, or making it part of my bedtime routine at the end of the day, was a fun exercise to do. What I discovered by this simple action was how tensely I held my body throughout the day as well as how much energy it took to keep all those muscles tight. The sense of relief of letting go when collapsing and letting gravity hold me was comforting, as I felt supported and held in such a calming way. It helped me to identify parts of the muscle groups in my body of which I had been totally unaware. Gradually, I was able to use this awareness to develop my skill of exploring the physicality of emotional sensations, and to start to identify where emotions manifested themselves in my body, still part of my ongoing mindfulness practice.

My perception and awareness of the world about me, how my body responded to events and emotions and the thoughts that dominated my mind were beginning to change. Maybe it was worth continuing with the mindfulness programme and the associated home practice, even when it all felt like very hard and emotionally painful work. How I saw myself and my place in the world was being turned upside-down and it was scary... I wonder what the next session is about!

Week 5: Being with difficulty

At this time, I was facing so many challenges in my life, possible retirement and negotiating the benefit system that did not understand the variable and fluctuating nature of ME/CFS. On top of all that, I was struggling with the symptoms of a cold. I wanted to run away from the whole lot, and not stay and face the stress, anxiety and grief that was hurting me. I did not want to face any more difficulty this week!

After the arrival and movement practice and the following inquiry process, I felt calmer. We were then introduced to the Chinese finger trap, and playing with this simple puzzle was one pivotal point in my mindfulness journey. As a nurse, I had always learnt by doing, and when inserting my index fingers into each end of this woven bamboo tube, the instinctive action was to pull my fingers out of the tube, which only tightened the trap around them. Though counterintuitive, by pushing the fingers together, the trap was loosened and my fingers were free!

The learning I took away from this practical exercise was not to fight or avoid difficult situations as running may not be helpful. Facing the fear is potentially a way to work with stressful and anxious situations. I realized that I was keeping myself busy as a distraction. The fruitless energy I was using to procrastinate and avoid difficult and scary situations was significantly contributing to the boom-and-bust cycle that had trapped me. I am still caught out by that trap even now!

Another exercise that we did in the session was to outline how I recognized the effect on my body, thoughts, feelings and behaviours when facing difficult or challenging times. Using the Threat/protective mode of the emotional regulation systems, the behaviours were easy to outline and were all examples of escaping or avoiding challenging situations, such as watching endless TV and neglecting caring for myself by grazing/snacking mainly on junk food.

Identifying bodily sensations was still a major challenge, but I started to explore and identify how tension manifested itself in my body and recognized the heavy sensation in my chest accompanied by a turbulent sensation in the upper part of my stomach, a tightness in my throat and my respirations becoming shallow and slower. The emotions, so familiar to me, were sadness, feeling alone, being very impatient with others, and feeling very guilty, though I did not know why. My dominant thoughts were that I was not trying hard enough to get better from the disabling symptoms that I was experiencing, the pain, fatigue and cognitive fog. I must try harder!

I wondered whether self-punishing thoughts went against the principles of mindfulness. I was doing my best to take advantage of all that was being offered in order to feel better, but perhaps I was not being kind and gentle with myself? I found this quote in the handouts we used that made sense of what I was becoming gradually aware of, the goal is to be aware and have choices:

> The goal of mindfulness is not to feel better. The goal is to open up yourself to the vitality of the moment, and thus *have a greater opportunity to make choices that enable you to move more effectively toward what you value.* (Hayes and Smith 2005) [my emphasis]

This week, the home practice suggested trying the sitting meditation without the guided CD, but I still was very apprehensive about making the change. I kept losing focus during the sitting practice, and there were times when I felt bored as the pace of the meditation dialogue was too slow. An unexpected thought occurred to me! Perhaps I was missing the aim of *being* mindful. The familiar words of the guided meditation started to take on new meaning and I realized that I had been *doing* breathing, instead of *being* with my breath. Previously, I was checking out that I was 'doing the breathing properly', but now I focused on how the breath was moving through my body, the feeling of it entering my nostrils, the coolness of my breath at the top of my palate, and then a sensation of dryness as the breath moved to the back of my throat and over the back of my soft palate.

When a coughing fit occurred, I tried to 'stay with the irritation' at the back of my throat but could not stop the coughing. Rather than disrupt my meditation totally, I dealt with the cough, then refocused on my breathing for a short time. How interesting to reflect that in earlier stages I had seen coughing as an interruption, rather than as part of my experience in which I might allow myself to explore how and where the cough could be felt in my body. When focusing on sounds in the environment, it was a delight to realize that I could hear the clock ticking in the next room, the silence in between each tick, the lack of street noise and the glass in the window cracking as it was expanding in the warmth of the beautiful sunshine. I could also hear myself swallowing when attempting to stave off a coughing fit. These were experiences that I had never paid attention to before.

My thoughts were interesting, and I did try to just observe them as they arose and not get involved with them; but I was aware of an aspect of my thinking – how often I considered my daily job list, prioritizing each task and deciding what needed to be done first when the meditation was over. These thoughts were accompanied by a feeling of being pressurized and overwhelmed, and a sense of anxiety and panic. I realized that I tended to beat myself up because I was not achieving as much in the day as I once did. I was even able to identify the physical sensations that accompany these thoughts, a knot in my middle belly, a heaviness in my left chest, with a feeling of needing to move and get going and do something – maybe that was called impatience? And was I wasting my time by meditating?

With all these new discoveries and experiences, I was beginning to enjoy practising mindfulness and that it was not so much of a chore as at the beginning of the programme. I hoped that the benefit of continuing my practice would manifest itself, rather than stressing out about whether jobs were getting done.

The one exercise that I kept forgetting to do when feeling really stressed, uptight or anxious was the coping pause strategy. I was beginning to be aware that continually grazing and snacking on unhealthy foods as a soothing behaviour was not helpful, and I was gaining weight dramatically. However, there had been so many challenges to explore that I could forgive myself for not attempting all of the home practices.

I had spent a lot of time thinking and reflecting during this week and concluded that there were several 'difficult' feelings and emotions lurking around, the main emotions being fear and regret. It had been suggested enough times that the only way to work with and through these painful emotions is gently to stay present with all experiences, including those unwanted emotions or sensations. It was about *taking the risk to stay with my feelings and not move away*. How was I going to do that? I then remembered how in last week's meditation practice, the words 'held and supported' came to mind. Perhaps I was telling myself that I *can* hold and support myself to face these scary emotions and sensations but was not aware of the implication of this introspection until now. Perhaps I do have the kindness, gentleness and compassion to care for myself when facing fear, which often paralyses me. What is interesting is the synchronicity of my life experience then and the next steps in the programme. There was so much I had to learn, and I was determined to continue with my practice even after the programme ended. I had some sense of hope. I did not yet know the plan of how I would go about continuing my mindfulness practice.

Week 6: Thoughts aren't facts

As soon as I arrived at this session, the title of the session, written on the whiteboard, grabbed my attention and the meaning of this strap line hit me between the eyes like a brick: Thoughts are just mental events, *not facts*! [my emphasis].

Even though I had chosen to study neurophysiology as a module in my first degree, I had never considered that the thoughts which were continually eating away at me during the day were just a neurophysiological activity. My mind was spinning with the revelation of this new idea as we commenced the session with an arrival and sitting practice, supposedly focusing on our body, breath, sounds and thoughts, and followed by the group inquiry. I found it impossible to be aware of my experience during this practice, as my logical mind was in overdrive, trying not to lose the impact of this significant 'ah-ha' moment. I wanted to keep it close to me, and not let it go or risk its meaning fading with the arrival of other thoughts. It was a time when I did not need a flashing PowerPoint presentation of thoughts moving relentlessly across my mind's eye!

We then considered a collection of thoughts that are common to people living with fatigue and other pain conditions during their 'bust' cycle. The highly negative and judgemental thoughts really resonated not just with me, but with others in the group. For me, it had been a difficult week with loads of unfinished forms and unrealistic expectations and challenges from overbearing bureaucracy, so facing up to and working with very challenging thoughts and emotions was quite painful.

Our personal thoughts during the different phases of the boom-and-bust cycle were then explored and how these thoughts could affect our experience of living with ME/CFS. In a strange way, it was reassuring to hear that other people had very similar thoughts to me during these times. During the following week, it was easy to make a note of my thoughts and the effect they had on me during the 'bust' phase, as that was how I was experiencing how my life was then. My dominant thoughts were 'I am so lazy', 'I am useless' and 'I am a failure', resulting in feeling exhausted and hopeless and realizing that operating from the Threat/Drive emotional regulation system was very familiar.

I really worked hard to explore where I felt these emotions in my body and came up with a list: a deflated feeling in my chest; stooped posture; head lowered, shoulders hunched; a knot in my upper abdominal region; teeth clenched; a tightness in my throat, conscious of letting out a low growl. What did I feel like doing? Screaming, yelling and crying! What an uptight and angry person I was! And that amount of energy I was wasting battling the emotional torment!

I thought back to a time that I felt energized, which I now accept is the 'boom' part of the cycle, and a familiar thought that sprang to mind was 'This is easy. I have tons of energy!' and feeling energetic, happy, sociable, enthusiastic, organized and clear-headed. I remembered a sense of lightness in my chest, and energy in my body, with a feeling of recovered strength in my arms and legs. My prevailing thought was I must get going whilst the going is good! My goal was to complete my never-ending job list before I ran out of energy. What a recipe for disaster! My thoughts and resulting unrealistic activity from the Drive system of emotional regulation was fuelling my boom-and-bust cycle.

However, this week saw a significant turning point in my mindfulness journey. After realizing that I saw thoughts as real facts, rather than treating them as mental events, I knew I needed more time to explore and challenge my natural and automatic thinking. The crunch came when I concluded that if thoughts are just mental events, maybe the critical and punitive thoughts which plagued me were not true? I had always tried to be kind and compassionate towards others, but why was I so judgemental, harsh, uncompassionate and angry towards myself? I would not purposely treat or speak to anyone else in such a way. This revelation, along with the regular invitation in the guided mindfulness meditation to be 'kindly curious', was key to trying to choose responses, thoughts and actions that were more compassionate, patient and kinder towards myself.

I considered what I could say to myself when those negative thoughts were invading my mind and impacting on how I felt and dealt with the exacerbation of ME/CFS symptoms:

'There's no day gone in next week!' (a favourite saying of my mother)
'I wouldn't be so hard/judgemental/harsh on someone else.'
'I need some kindness now, so just be gentle [with myself].'

There were some strategies that I could choose to do when feeling so bruised and battered. One was to prioritize, plan and break up challenging tasks into much smaller tasks by making a list and not setting unrealistic deadlines on completing each step. The other plan, which developed from the habit releaser exercise from this session, was to engage in activities that tapped into the Soothing mode of the emotional regulation systems. There were so many activities that I had not done for years that I used to really enjoy – knitting, jigsaw puzzles, sketching, colouring and birdwatching, all of which did not tax my energy levels at the time. I tried the knitting and really enjoyed making a scarf, the rhythmic action of the wool around the needles was soothing, and the sense of achievement as my scarf grew longer was gratifying. I even adapted my knitting technique so that I could knit when lying on the sofa whilst resting.

I now allow myself permission to do what I need to do to take care of myself more frequently, especially when having a setback. Slowly, my self-concept is changing – I am no longer *useless* or a *failure*, but someone who continues learning to adapt to living with the symptoms of ME/CFS. Life has become more enjoyable, despite living with a long-term condition, and the adage is true... When one door closes, another one opens!

I continued with my mindfulness meditation practice that week and missed it when I did not manage to fit in a formal practice one day. I was really enjoying using my sitting stool and exploring my thoughts, emotions, my environment, sounds heard and bodily sensations without the use of a guided meditation to lead me. I appreciated the freedom to stop, explore and focus in more depth, whatever came to the forefront of my attention, rather than feeling that I was not following the guidance properly when curiosity overcame me.

I was beginning to understand that mindfulness doesn't mean getting annoyed because I was not *doing* the exercises 'properly' – that judgemental thought came from me and, after all, it was only a mental event. Mindfulness was about being in the here and now and being curious and aware of where my mind, thoughts and consciousness went. I was starting to be gentler with myself and also with other people and started to recognize what I could and couldn't control. I wondered where this journey would eventually lead me... I was coming to the end of this programme and felt rather sad and anxious about that. I was just beginning my mindfulness journey.

Week 7: Taking care of myself

It was strange how this last session panned out. I thought I would be very sad that the programme had finished, but the activities helped me realize how much I had learnt, how my approach to living was changing and that I still had that determination to continue with my mindfulness practice.

We considered how to take care of ourselves during the next month, when we would have a review session with a clinical specialist. The first task was to develop a daily plan that included a range of activities to help us decide what needed doing, especially in the face of feeling low in mood, tired or challenged by discouraging thoughts. The important thing for me was to include nourishing activities that would help me to feel alive and present in my daily plan, as at that time only jobs that needed to be done were on my list, hence continuing the habit of being a 'doer' rather than giving space for just 'being'. Some nourishing activities were not possible to add to my daily routine, such as swimming in the sea or walking along a beach, but just being outside, engaging with nature and observing the changing season.

Accepting that there are aspects of my life that I cannot change, how could I deal with those draining activities that still needed doing? These were jobs around the house, socializing with others, worrying about my future and battling with my unreliable cognitive skills when reading, writing or making telephone calls. First, it was obvious that I needed to continue with regular meditation practice, especially the anchoring pause, so that at these demanding times, I could automatically ground myself when feeling overwhelmed or outpaced. There was also a new strategy, developing my sense of curiosity that I was just beginning to practise. I wondered how that telephone call would turn out if I am nice to the other person at the end of the line. Will that make any difference to the outcome of a challenging and much dreaded task for me? Tentatively, I was finding out that the outcome was usually positive for me, and I was more likely to achieve what I needed without energy being wasted on being anxious and fearful. It was also interesting to listen to the brief conversation of the other person, helping me to realize that they were not an ogre but a person, who was often doing a thankless task.

We also thought about planning what to do if we found that our symptoms of ME/CFS were worsening. Rather than going into panic mode, I planned that I would be gentle with myself by adjusting the levels of physical and cognitive activities and breaking larger tasks into smaller steps. I also planned to ask for help, something that I had not done before, but when I did test it out I was amazed at the offer of meals and support that were given. Another thing was to allow myself to do enjoyable and nourishing activities during this time, whether it just be something as simple as looking out of the window from my bed watching the weather and the clouds drift by.

At the end of the programme, I was able to accept that a setback is likely to be part of the course, but I didn't need to beat myself up about it. After all, I am living with a chronic condition and I plan to live as well as possible with it, rather than the continual daily fight, and to be mindful of my fatigue, pain, emotions and thoughts during this time. Another strategy was to plan to consider positive events that occurred each day during this time to balance my tendency to sink into the depths of despair.

Making mindful decisions was becoming more of a habit in my daily life as the questions I so frequently heard on the guided meditations often arose when I felt that I was struggling in a situation:

- 'What do I need to do right now?'
- 'How can I best look after myself right now?'
- 'What does my body need now?'

Often, it is reminding myself to stop and spend time doing a nourishing activity or attending to my physiological needs, such as having a drink or a short rest. I was learning to be more flexible with my daily 'to do' list, by moving jobs to tomorrow, the day after or even next week to allow time to nurture myself.

I felt confident that I would be able to sustain my mindfulness meditation practice during the next month as I was enjoying exploring the use of a meditation timer app and sitting on my meditation stool, which now I was finding comfortable. I was fascinated allowing myself to pay attention to whatever arose in my consciousness – thoughts, bodily sensations, emotional feelings, sounds and even smells, a sense that I seemed to totally neglect. A new sensation this week was that I was feeling hungry. It was an empty feeling in my upper belly, like a funnel emptying. How could I have ever been unaware of that sensation?

I was still not using the anchoring and coping pauses regularly but found an app for my phone that gave me random reminders during the day, and over time these short practices became a natural way of coping with stressful situations.

What brought me to the course in the first place was wanting to learn how to banish the symptoms of ME/CFS by finding that 'magic wand' which would make all my debilitating symptoms disappear. Instead, I have been introduced to mindfulness practice and been shown the tools that will help me to live *well* with ME/CFS. The inspiring words by the writer and philosopher Alfred D'Souza sum up my experience of the adapted MBCT programme:

> For a long time, it had seemed to me that life was about to begin – real life. But there was always some obstacle in the way, something to be gotten through first, some unfinished business, time to be served, a debt to be paid. Then life would begin. At last, it dawned on me that these obstacles were my life.

What has changed for me?

After the MBCT programme and continuing practising mindfulness, I have observed numerous changes in myself:

- Kinder and gentler with myself:
  I found that the repeated reminders to be 'kind and gentle' with myself in

the guided meditations meant that I started to incorporate this compassionate approach to my daily life. Asking myself 'What do I need now?' or 'What do I need to do now?' reminded me to take care of myself and to meet any physical, emotional or mental need that once I would have ignored.

- More content with my life:
  Being able to recognize and value the pleasant events that regularly happen in my daily life, no matter how trivial, means that I have a more balanced outlook on life. I am more of a 'cup half full' person now, rather than a 'half empty' one. I am able to see the world (despite all the dreadful events that are happening now) in a more positive light. I am learning to choose how to react/respond to what 'life throws at me' by being aware of my thoughts and emotions and where I feel them in my body. Consequently, I feel more in control of my life.

Developing the attitudinal factors of mindfulness

The seven attitudinal factors of mindfulness (Kabat-Zinn 2013) provided a framework which has helped me to focus and reflect on my evolving practice of mindfulness. The seven factors are:

1. Non-judging:
   I realized that it was me who had always been my harshest critic, and by believing those powerful negative thoughts, my self-confidence and self-esteem were significantly affected. Being kinder with myself means that I am also less critical and judgemental of others as well.

2. Patience:
   Because I am kinder and gentler with myself, I now have more patience with both myself and others. I now see that making mistakes or wandering up a blind alley can be used as a learning opportunity. How could I do things differently? It does not warrant feeling frustrated, angry or impatient.

3. Acceptance:
   I have always been driven to be perfect in all aspects of my life. Keeping up the standards was exhausting, but a gradual acceptance of myself and realizing that I am not a 'failure', but someone who is living bravely with a long-term condition that often affects how I am able to live each day, has been a relief. As a result, I waste less energy regretting my past or worrying about the future, so have more energy to live and enjoy each day. I accept that there will be times when there will be a relapse, but I do not fight or get so angry with myself when it does happen but take

note of what I need at that time. There is a sense of freedom that comes with accepting myself.

4. Non-striving:
   Practising mindfulness regularly means more time spent being and so much less time in aimless doing, and experiencing fewer episodes of the boom-and-bust cycle. Throughout this chapter, I have emphasized the words *doing* and *being* so I could see when being mindful was becoming part of my way of life. It appears that I did not recognize the mode of Being until at least after Session 6! Being takes practice! Williams and Penman (2011) outlined the seven characteristics of Doing and Being modes of mind. I was continually operating from the Doing mode, striving to live successfully, and forgetting to care for myself, in preference to the endless cycle of maintaining standards, completing deadlines, accepting ever-increasing workloads and unrealistic expectations. I was certainly living in the fast lane and continually felt panicky and overwhelmed by mounting lists of jobs to do.

5. Trust:
   As a result of practising mindfulness regularly, I now recognize, take heed and trust my inner wisdom, a gift that I never realized that I possessed. I had always sought and relied on the advice of others, who sometimes did not have my best interests at heart.

6. Letting go:
   I think the letting go was the hardest bit for me to work on. I had so many regrets – regrets for the life and activity levels I once had, the lost identity as a nurse and lecturer in higher education, and the unfinished PhD due to my 'brain fog'. However, as I started to let go of some of these regrets, I began to find new fulfilling adventures that I could respond to and that accommodated my changing lifestyle due to living with a chronic and fatiguing condition. It was also helped by a better understanding of how to pace myself effectively. I acknowledge the skills that I gained in my former career and use them in ways that I never envisaged. It is interesting how life is turning out as a result of letting go!

7. Beginner's mind:
   I have always possessed this attitudinal factor of mindfulness, and the sense of curiosity embedded in my mindfulness practice has meant that I continue to learn new things about myself and the world around me.

How did these dramatic changes happen?

To tell you the truth, I have no idea *how* these changes in my life happened! I did make a commitment to complete the regular home practice and written exercises and reflected on my experiences in a journal. I found participating in the inquiry process and sharing and listening to others' experiences in each session was a beneficial learning opportunity and that very old behaviours and thoughts were changing. It was an exciting time of growth.

The learning and development from mindfulness is a continuous process, and by no means have I reached the end of the road in my journey, but that is the exciting part of this lifelong journey. Looking ahead, even when I become physically frail due to the inevitable ageing process and unable to do much, I will be always able to practise just being in the here and now.

Encouraged to be curious about my mindfulness experience and asking myself 'What am I experiencing right now?', the helpless, timid, fearful, anxious, detached and tearful 'victim' of a long-term condition has all but disappeared. Instead of living with the multitude of negative emotions, thoughts and behaviours, I now try to live each day mindfully. What I have learnt from the mindfulness journey can be summarized by my favourite quote by an unknown author: 'Replace fear of the unknown with curiosity.'

Chapter 19

Creating and Sustaining a Team

- Mindfulness practice as the basis of training
- A specific group with specific needs
- Clinician training
- Understanding self-management
- Ongoing clinician support and supervision
- Considerations of working within an institution

Mindfulness practice as the basis of training

This chapter will consider the therapist's own practice along with some of the particularities of this clinical area and the standards and training requirements of both the clinical field and contemporary mindfulness good practice.

The nature of a mindfulness-based programme, of whatever flavour, is that the practitioner is using mindfulness, firstly for themselves in their own life and work and secondly as the basis for their interactions. A hallmark of this approach is that progress is not defined by how well one meditates but how much more happiness, curiosity, patience, etc. one develops and how this can support the life we want to lead, which seems to take it very much beyond a clinical intervention into the way life is lived regardless of health status.

The requirements of the British Association of Mindfulness-Based Approaches (BAMBA) are that practitioners have a formal practice including daily formal practice and regular retreats (UK Network of Mindfulness Teacher Training Organisations 2015). Of course, it is possible to see this as something for working hours and then to feel squeezed in work time to do this. However, this misses an opportunity for mindfulness to be part of the clinician's life and to support every aspect of it. Which in turn supports the group's lived experience and takes it beyond a technique aimed at managing health.

To teach according to UK best practice guidelines, we need to appreciate mindfulness not as a toolbox, but as a whole way of looking at the world.

Mindfulness can only be understood from the inside out. It is not one more cognitive-behavioural technique to be deployed in a behaviour change paradigm, but a way of being and a way of seeing that has profound implications for understanding the nature of our own minds and bodies, and for living life as if it really mattered. (Kabat-Zinn 2013)

This involves exploring one's own experience and developing this with guidance from teachers and fellow travellers and inhabiting our experience and sharing with others; as mindfulness-based therapists, clinicians, teachers, whatever we call ourselves, we have to work within our own humanity, perhaps summed up by these words from Mary Oliver's poem 'Wild Geese': 'Tell me about despair, yours, and I will tell you mine.'

Figure 19.1 describes how this feels – a mindfulness-based approach is not just what we do in the group, it echoes through all that we do. I may find myself intentionally using a mindfulness-based approach, for example in an individual therapy or supervision session when there is a sense of anxiety or feeling fraught and vexed – to pause, find feet, breathe, let the mind wander and gently inhabit the senses, then ask what feels important or where the challenge is felt in the body. I may have had a bad night's sleep with a worry about a family member, and need to ground and energize myself through a short walking practice before starting work. Then make sure I have a rest at lunchtime so I can be present for the group in the afternoon. A formal daily practice and regular retreats and connection with others in my personal life who have a practice and who share delights and challenges is crucial. As time goes by, the more I am convinced this is a community endeavour; how can we let go of stress, worry and isolation without a safe place to go into? Equally, access to more experienced practitioners is motivating and supportive.

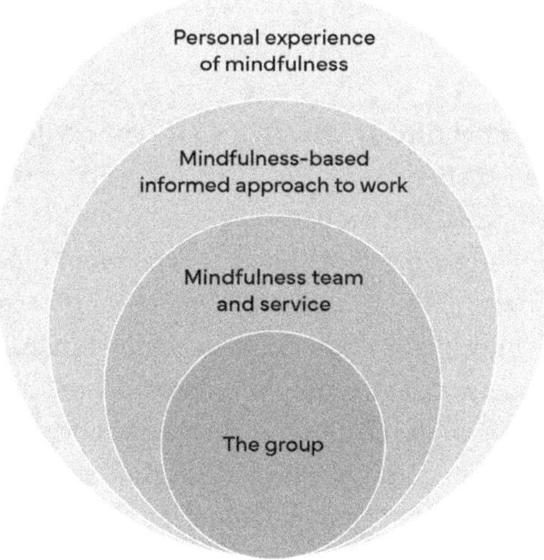

Figure 19.1 A clinician's mindfulness-based practice

A specific group with specific needs

This course is an adaptation and not a primary course; we have all trained in one of the standard courses and, as described in chapter 1, the adaptations we have made have been carefully considered with feedback and work with our participants (Crane et al. 2021). For the first six years of teaching, the Bangor 'hybrid' curriculum was used with a form of MBCT using the cognitive therapy evidence base in ME/CFS with support from Christina Surawy's work (Surawy et al. 2005) and supervision from Christina in developing the programme. Then experiencing other curricula, such as the MBSR (Santorelli et al. 2017) and Breathworks (Burch and Penman 2013) programmes, was separate to this and done in collaboration with an Improving Access to Psychological Therapies service and a Breathworks teacher. Having the space and professional freedom to do this was an important part of being able to develop. This meant working closely with clinical supervisors, the team and team leaders always holding the intention that we were there to offer patients support with living better with their health condition.

Working within a particular speciality requires understanding, firstly, of universal struggles and joys and how mindfulness practices allow us to engage wholeheartedly with life and the 'full catastrophe' therein; and then, of the specific challenges a group of people may have. Even (especially?) if the practitioner has a personal experience of the condition, as this will not be the 'full range' of experience that can arise and there needs to be a curious awareness of a myriad of experiences brought by each person within the field of practice. The feedback from our evaluation was that this very particular understanding was useful, supportive and powerful. This resonates with some research that showed the therapeutic alliance was a more powerful moderator of distress reduction than therapist skill (Bisseling et al. 2019).

Understanding and experiencing self-management

While having direct experience of ME/CFS, fibromyalgia and Long Covid is not a prerequisite for working with people with those conditions, having experience of self-management strategies most likely is. The mindfulness programme is targeted at people who find the self-management approach challenging and do not need more information, but do need understanding of the challenge self-management presents. For example, a common self-management tool is to keep an activity diary (see chapter 14), but unless one has been attempted personally, it is hard to understand how challenging this can be, what it shows and what it doesn't show. For example, emotional high energy is unlikely to be recorded in an activity diary as it might be happening while one is doing something seemingly of lower intensity, such making a salad or watching TV.

Similarly, with scheduling rest and working within baselines of activity, but understanding this from the 'inside' may help. We may not use baselines or set goals because of health limits; it is a way of doing things that may enhance and enable our personal lives.

For example, I am currently walking a long-distance path with a friend; we noticed that the published routes and descriptions were in 12- to 15-mile chunks. We realized that we were not able to do that, partly due to fitness and also because we started in November and there wasn't enough daylight, so we have worked out that our baseline at the moment is five to eight miles and have restructured the route, but not completely, as we hope that as the days get longer (and perhaps we get fitter) we can manage longer sections. How many times in life are we presented with something that is 'the way to do it' when in actual fact it is *a* way to do it, and other ways are available?

Progress is marked in self-management not by the absence or amelioration of symptoms, but by the achievement of realistic and meaningful goals that are reviewed, appreciated and applauded on the way – each step is valid in its own right and may open up new perspectives, experiences and new ideas and therefore new goals. In a health setting, this is about creating health from where the individual is now in a life that each individual personally curates. While this is the goal of a self-management approach to health, it is much larger than that, it is how a meaningful life can be experienced. For clinicians, spending time on one's own goals and definitely appreciating and applauding them, perhaps with some support from a coach or therapist or (even better) like-minded friends, can be personally rewarding but will also thicken up one's clinical practice.

A personalized goal-focused approach is being clear about what I want to do, thinking about what is realistic and marking success by the achievement of those, but also enjoying the process. I may never get to the end of the path, but so far, the five-mile chunks have lit up my winter once a month and I have learnt things I didn't know were there to be learnt and enjoyed – bird names, map features, historical events, things about my friend, and so on. This may lead me to other places, reading about a particular part of history, booking a week in a town, walking in a different place. By appreciating each step and then looking to see where I want to go next, the process of working within the goal is meaningful and fulfilling and creates the conditions for what happens next. If I made it solely about getting to the end of the path, I may miss the other opportunities and experiences. Embodying and valuing this as a way to live may not be shared directly, but attempts to prevent the approach being something 'done to' the person.

Progress in a mindfulness-based approach is marked by an increased capacity for self-care, self-compassion, acceptance and friendliness to experience. We and our patients can step out of survival mode and into living. It is often said that these qualities are 'caught not taught', and it is the embodied presence of the practitioner, showing up with their humanity, flaws and all, and offering themselves and others these qualities over and over again, that allows this to emerge.

Mindfulness training for clinicians

Before looking at what the training and practice looks like, let's listen to what our participants say about the experience of learning mindfulness in a specialist service.

- First, about the specifics of being in a group with others who have similar health conditions, including one of the facilitators:

  'It helped you to see…we're having a bad day today or they're having a really bad day today; you could work it through with each other, how we are gonna get ourselves out of this to a level, so we are not booming and busting any more. That was quite important. I was a push through and ended up out of it, that is not actually helpful long-term to live. I felt like when I started I was surviving and by the end it felt more like I was living and that was a really important change.'

  'It is good to see how other people are coping, some of the things you think are just of you, you then realize everyone is doing that, so you do learn, you learn by listening. When you do realize that some people are coping with going to work, that was helpful for me because I think I thought that the rest of my life is gone, then you realize some people are coping with managing their families, managing jobs, that is quite encouraging.'

  'I didn't feel anyone judged me and everyone was given a voice; it was nice to have someone there who 100% gets it, you can sort of kind of understand, but until you've walked in those shoes it's really difficult, even some of the home work, she came back and said I couldn't do it this week. If Rhonda can't do it we're alright.' [Rhonda, experienced patient involved in the group]

  'I'm not sure about going to one where it's open to everyone…unless you have walked through it you don't quite get it. You can be tired or have a bad day, and having a bad day is a relatable thing, but being able to walk into the room and "Oh, you know what, my legs just ain't happening today" and everyone goes, "Yeah, I've had that day." You don't have to explain it before you understand it. You can just say that's the thing it is. Definitely much better within the ME/CFS bubble.'

- How the team worked together, from a conversation in a focus group:

  A: 'I like how Fiona and Pete worked together; it seemed quite relaxed, good.'

  B: 'It is not rehearsed, it wasn't too formal.'

  A: 'It felt like we were all there together.'

  C: 'They were part of it, not looking from the outside in.'

  D: 'It was human.'

  C: 'There was no us and them.'

- Being within a specialist service:

  'I was off work at the start of it, and by the end of it I was back in work. It was a medical appointment that I needed to go to, to take care of myself. If it was just a group in a village hall, I wouldn't be allowed off work and I wouldn't have got as much from it. I wouldn't have the experiences of all the other people in the room that had the same condition as me. We have all experienced it in different ways. The fact that it was a medical appointment allowed me space in my day to come, which didn't take further energy by having to go in the evening. It just gave me a bit of permission to go being a medical appointment. Pete and Fiona work with people with this condition every single day, it felt safer than if it was with a general mindfulness teacher.'

  'The thing about these courses is how do you know the teacher knows what they are doing? I think it's been really good, I think at least half of what's been good about it is being with the other people.'

  'I would have been more apprehensive going to a general mindfulness. Because this was a ME/CFS thing, I was a lot more open-minded and willing to attempt it.'

  'I did some online CBT stuff before attending this. I had to take some time off work and the doctor said one of the things you need to do is CBT for your mood. One thing that stood out to me then was that one of the sayings was "if your mind says you can't do it, just do it". I thought if I haven't got the energy, if I have got fatigue I can't physically do it. The CBT stuff was written not for CFS/ME. Most of the stuff was general mindfulness and didn't cater for those difficult things. This course did that and boosted my knowledge on the things CBT didn't teach me. So it helped with what I need to do and what I can't physically do. Having the people around you that you can learn from, Fiona and Pete that you can learn from.'

So how do we get to this? A group of people who understand, encourage and support each other, give each other hope? Clinicians being able to be part of it, yet being professionals, and being specialists within a particular field with a detailed and deep knowledge of a particular type of condition? The latter perhaps partly comes from years of experience and ongoing immersion and training within the field, but also I feel comes from a mindfulness practice and inherent features of this 'way of being' required when working with health conditions when 'nothing more can be done' and there are no simple solutions the clinician can impart to the patient. The attitudinal foundations can take us a long way: curiosity; non-judgement; beginner's mind; patience; kindness immediately spring to mind within the above exchanges.

Training and sustaining mindfulness teachers

The British Association of Mindfulness-Based Approaches (BAMBA) works to good practice guidelines (UK Network of Mindfulness Teacher Training Organisations 2015), and while not a requirement for employment in the NHS, this has been the guiding principle for the training within the service. An apprenticeship model supplemented by external training and supervision has been developed and supported. Therapists need to have their own practice, and this is then used to reflect on teaching and the needs of the group. This is also how the team sustains and supports itself through shared practice days and time to reflect and develop. Volunteer patient facilitators can work at where they feel they can today, offering a lived experience of the practice and speaking from where they are today in the groups.

It is anticipated that this adapted mindfulness-based programme could be used by clinicians with mindfulness training but with less contextual support. But that they would require clinical supervision as well as mindfulness-based supervision and be trained in (and have access to ongoing CPD) current thinking on chronic pain, fatigue and post-viral sequalae as well as the transdiagnostic rehabilitative (self-management) approach which would make it applicable to working with other specific groups (e.g. Long Covid patients; arthritis, etc.). Places to access this include the British Pain Society, Pain Management SIG and the British Association of Clinicians in ME/CFS (BACME). The British Pain Society has developed clinical competencies in pain management.

For specialist clinicians working within a fatigue or pain-management service, then considering how to add in a mindfulness-based approach to individuals or groups of patients will mean evaluating the resources and time they have for training as well as the commitment to self-practice. There are various routes to this but the BAMBA guidelines give clear guidance and pathways to training.

Service examples of training

Our service has used a mixture of training methods, including Master's level accreditation, standalone retreat-based training, workshop training opportunities, co-teaching, supervision and apprenticeship-style training. This has evolved, and we feel that each clinician needed to have their own practice and find a way to training that suited their personal circumstances.

The apprenticeship model works well as a starting point; clinicians can start by doing the course for themselves, and support the group with emails, managing enquiries and hosting the video platform. Currently, we have three staff doing the course for themselves, and we run a separate breakout room for them to discuss their home practice as well as for some time at the end. They are directed to specific reading material and can have individual supervision. If they wish to take this further, they are first very much encouraged to find a mindfulness course for themselves (in their own time) and develop their practice in their own way. They can then come to the group and be involved in active reflection and lead short sessions with support with inquiry. Further training will be required before they can hold and run the group, but we find that as time goes by practitioners become more autonomous and have a variety of voices and approaches.

Patient volunteers go through a similar process, and they can be involved to whatever extent feels comfortable, from sharing experience of living with fatigue to joining in the inquiry, reading poems and leading practices. Of the co-contributors to this book, Sarah Nearney has gone on to full training in teaching, has developed the movement practice and can teach a full course. She is also starting to offer mindfulness within her professional clinical field, palliative care. Rhonda Knight actively participates in the groups, supports home practice reflection and mindful activity and shares poems and thoughts as well as contributing to the handouts and literature. She has also been involved in staff training locally and nationally.

Supervision

Mindfulness-based supervision is a place to integrate theoretical learning, experiences in facilitating mindfulness-based practitioners (MBPs) and the relationship between personal and professional practice. It is fundamental to our approach:

Mindfulness-based supervision is key to supporting Mindfulness teachers' learning and development, and for the emergent field of MBPs to maintain standards and integrity. (Evans cited in Crane et al. 2021, p.156)

Following one's personal interest and experience is part of the joy of working within a mindfulness-based approach. The experiential and inquiring nature of the approach means there is a constant development and change while maintaining the integrity of the delivered mindfulness programme of whatever flavour. Each facilitator will have their own style and each group will have its own personality, and supervision can develop, challenge and support practice. In a specific programme like ours, it may not be possible to have a facilitator who has direct experience of the nuances of the service or the clinical population, so supervision is a place to reflect, consider and develop. If one is the sole or lead mindfulness practitioner in a team, then having a place to consider, reflect and also have feedback on the approach and how mindfulness is unfolding in a new setting is essential. Additional clinical supervision is required, to maintain the ingredients, and peers can support this further.

Clinicians supporting each other

Before each group session we meet and discuss the session, the theme and anything we might need to think about for specific participants; we discuss how our practice is, how we are and how the theme of the session is alive for us right now. For example, Session 4, the theme of staying present within the constant flux of our experience – how is this happening right now? And how does this approach support us in our own particular circumstances? While we don't share the details of this in the group (unless it feels particularly appropriate), we are aware of how the other is feeling, and this has meant we have been able to keep working during some personally delicate times. This has meant at points one of us may lead the whole group, while the other is there as a presence to be involved in the unfolding inquiring nature of the group; at other times, there may be clear sharing of leading and holding.

Interestingly, like the participants who sometimes show up saying they don't feel great and may be very quiet, we often say we feel better by the end of a session, even if it's a two-hour Zoom call. This nurturing and care of each other has I think taught us to lean into the practice, to be curious and come back to beginner's mind, and also to acknowledge when sometimes we slip from this, when we are pushing ourselves to be a certain way, when we are exhausted and have no patience. Knowing when to take time out while also looking after the group.

By understanding each other's mindfulness practice, we can draw out nuances that may be helpful for the participants. For example, some of us do not like the instruction 'breathing into the toes' as it makes no anatomical sense; others fully feel it and have a different sense of this. This means we offer guidance that resonates with us individually and we hope meets the varying sensibilities of the group participants. This difference is sometimes discussed explicitly in the session that models diversity of experience and acceptance and disrupts the idea that there is a 'correct' way to 'do' mindfulness practice.

Working within an institution

In order to deliver a mindfulness programme within organizations such as the NHS, there are a number of factors that influence the group, including the evidence base and guidelines for the condition as well as the mindfulness-based therapy itself. Staff need not only to be available, but also to be resourced enough to teach because they are using their personhood intimately.

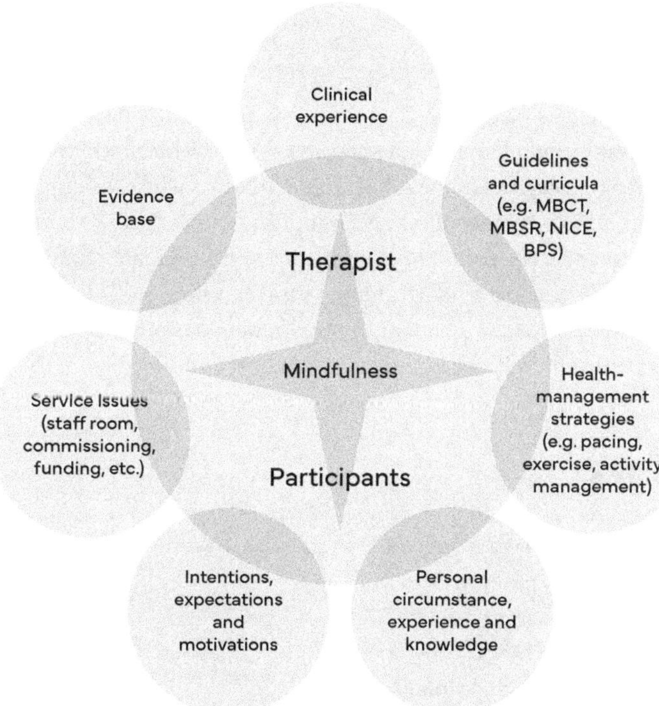

Figure 19.2 Components of running a mindfulness-based programme

Figure 19.2 represents what needs to be considered, and each service and practitioner and participant will have different experiences of each component, certainly course by course, but likely also session by session, and varying needs to be navigated delicately. The figure shows the ingredients of a mindfulness programme within a particular setting, and without each of these ingredients, the 'cake' will be different. The therapist will be holding all of this in the moment to a greater or lesser degree. While the participants won't have so much to do with the commissioning process and guidelines, the group will not exist in a specialist service without some work in both those domains. For the therapist, any one of those domains can impact on how we work. For example, the 2021 change in ME/CFS NICE guidance meant we considered the nature of the work and how we articulated this between ourselves and with the patient group. Personal circumstances can affect things too.

The box below gives an example of changes made by one clinician that enabled her to look after herself, look after her service and keep the mindfulness programme on the agenda but not overload herself. Going forward, there are likely to be other changes that mean the patients get a useful service and she does not burn herself out by trying to be all things to all people all the time.

A very experienced mindfulness-based clinician experienced significant health challenges and had staffing shortages. She did not feel able to continue running the full mindfulness course, so took a break while continuing to work clinically. Her health started to resolve while she committed to both her self-management and mindfulness practice with ongoing supervision and retreats. This folded into her individual clinical work and then she was able to start running shorter online courses (one hour for four weeks) to give a flavour of mindfulness to her participants and also build on the self-management work she was doing day to day.

SUMMARY

- In order to deliver a specific mindfulness-based programme clinicians or therapists need to have:
    - personal practice
    - an understanding and experience of the specific challenges participants will be experiencing.
- This takes personal commitment and requires the support of colleagues and the institution in which one works.
- UK guidelines require mindfulness practitioners to have clinical and mindfulness-based supervision and attend annual retreats as part of maintaining their practice.
- Practitioners also need to be aware of developments within the field and consider how and if this needs to be part of the mindfulness programme (see changes following 2021 NICE guidance change).

Summary of the Approach

This book is a description of how mindfulness-based cognitive therapy has been adapted for people living with fatiguing conditions that impact significantly on their lives. Ninety per cent of people in NHS clinics struggle to work or go to school. Coming to a diagnosis is difficult as there are no biomedical markers or tests or clarity about the mechanism so it is not possible to treat medically. After a lot of inconclusive investigations, people are often told they need to 'learn to live with it'.

A mindfulness-based approach came from conversations with patients who had been through the self-management programmes to help people manage but who were struggling with the reality of 'living with it'.

We started and trained with the MBCT and MBSR programmes with some adaptation to fatigue, based on work at the Oxford Mindfulness Centre (Surawy et al. 2005). After several years of running groups, and some evaluation, the programme developed. We identified there was a particular nuance to the practices and adaptations to delivery. For example, there was a need to focus on using the potentially restful nature of mindfulness practice by learning to 'stop' or 'pause'. This included emphasizing the unwinding of tension in the body and developing a compassionate awareness. This has enabled people being able to experiment with changing their approach to activity and rest.

The information in the session is reduced to manage fatigue, and the sessions are structured to be accessible to a range of cognitive and physical abilities. The fluctuating nature of the conditions means needs can vary from session to session. This is reflected in graded practices, a choice in handout, ways people can physically access the group.

The stories and quotes from people who have informed and reflected on the approach is woven throughout each chapter.

The process of implementation and the development within the fatigue and pain-management services is discussed including gaining 'top-down' and colleague buy-in and referral.

Training requirements are discussed in both directions: mindfulness teachers who need to understand more about fatigue and self-management approaches or clinicians who wish to develop a mindfulness-based approach.

The wider context is considered an essential part of the approach, for example the impact of and support required regarding employment, childcare and finance. I don't think it's coincidence that the other work stream I lead is employment concerns. I personally have a strong belief (and concern) that both mindfulness and self-management need to be aware of a 'self-improvement agenda' that puts all the work onto the person who is struggling; there needs to be a contextual approach that works with the social and economic situation – for example, if someone is struggling to hold on to a job and manage a family, then 'self-management', never mind meditation without explicitly addressing this, can make everything worse. Addressing practical concerns (and empowering people to address or support by advocating) needs to be there as part of the approach (Durocher et al. 2014).

Practices and PowerPoints referred to are available at fionamckechnie.co.uk

Resources

Fatiguing conditions

- British Association of Clinicians in ME/CFS: https://bacme.info
  A multi-disciplinary organization providing information, resources, education and networking opportunities to UK professionals to deliver high quality care to people living with ME/CFS.

- Action for ME: www.actionforme.org.uk

- ME Association: https://meassociation.org.uk

- *ME/CFS/PVFs: An Exploration of Key Clinical Issues* (12th edn) by C. Shepherd and A. Chaudhuri 2020 (ME Association)
  This is updated regularly and worth getting each time.

- NICE guidance – www.nice.org.uk/guidance
  See the up-to-date guides for ME/CFS, Long Covid, chronic pain, long-term health conditions. Current ones include:
  - NICE (2021a) *COVID 19 Rapid Guideline: Managing the Long-term Effects of COVID-19* [NG188]. Available at http://covid19-rapid-guideline-managing-the-longterm-effects-of-covid19-pdf-51035515742
  - NICE (2021b) Chronic *Pain (Primary and Secondary) in over 16s: Assessment of All Chronic Pain and Management of Chronic Primary Pain* [NG193]. Available at www.nice.org.uk/guidance/ng193
  - NICE (2021c) *Myalgic Encephalomyelitis (or Encephalopathy)/Chronic Fatigue Syndrome: Diagnosis and Management* [NG206]. Available at www.nice.org.uk/guidance/ng206

- Bristol ME Service has videos and information about ME and Long Covid: www.nbt.nhs.uk/our-services/a-z-services/bristol-me-service

- *Living with ME and Chronic Fatigue Syndrome* by Dr Gerald Coakley and Beverly Knops 2022 (Penguin Random House)

- *Fighting Fatigue* by Sue Pemberton 2009 (Hammersmith Press)

Mindfulness

- *Full Catastrophe Living: How to Cope with Stress, Pain and Illness Using Mindfulness Meditation* by Jon Kabat-Zinn 2013 (Hachette)

- *Living Well with Pain and Illness. The Mindful Way to Free Yourself from Suffering* by Vidyamala Burch 2008 (Pitakus)

- *Mindfulness for Health* by Vidyamala Burch and Danny Penman 2013 (Piatkus)

- Breathworks – Mindfulness and Compassion Training: www.breath-works-mindfulness.org.uk
  Resources, training and courses for mindfulness for pain, illness and stress.

- *Mindfulness: A Practical Guide to Finding Peace in a Frantic World* by Mark Williams and Danny Penman 2011 (Piatkus)

- Mindfulness: Finding Peace in a Frantic World: http://franticworld.com
  Website of authors Danny Penman, Mark Williams and Vidyamala Burch.

- *The Mindful Way through Depression* by Mark Williams, John Teasdale, Zindel Segal and Jon Kabat-Zinn 2007 (Guilford Press)
  Comes with a CD narrated by Jon Kabat-Zinn.

- *The Mindful Path to Self-compassion* by Christopher Germer 2009 (Guilford Press)

- *Radical Acceptance: Embracing your Life with the Heart of a Buddha* by Tara Brach 2003 (Rider Books)

- *The Wisdom of No Escape* by Pema Chodron 2004 (Element Books)

- *The Miracle of Mindfulness* by Thich Nhat Hanh 2008 (Rider Books)

Mindfulness teaching

- BAMBA – British Association of Mindfulness-Based Approaches: https://bamba.org.uk

- Mindfulness Network: www.mindfulness-network.org
  Provides training, supervision and retreats as well as networking.

- *Essential Resources for Mindfulness Teachers* by R.S. Crane, Karunavira and G.M. Griffith (eds.) 2021 (Routledge)

- *Mindfulness-Based Stress Reduction (MBSR) Authorized Curriculum Guide* by S.F. Santorelli, F. Meleo-Meyer, L. Koerbel and J. Kabat-Zinn 2017 (Center for Mindfulness in Medicine, Healthcare, and Society, University of Massachusetts Medical School)

- *Mindfulness-based Cognitive Therapy for Depression* by Z. Segal, M. Williams and J. Teasdale 2013 (Guilford)

- *Mindfulness-based Cognitive Therapy: Distinctive Features* by R.S. Crane 2017 (Routledge)

- *Mindfulness-based Interventions: Teaching Assessment Criteria (MBI-TAC)* by W. Kuyken, R. Hastings, J. Soulsby, C. Eames et al. 2021. Available at https://mbitac.bangor.ac.uk/documents/MBITACmanual0517.pdf

- *Mindfulness: Ancient Wisdom Meets Modern Psychology* by C. Feldman and W. Kuyken 2019 (Guilford)

- *Words that Touch: How to Ask Questions Your Body Can Answer – 12 Essential 'Clean Questions' for Mind/Body Therapists* by N. Pole 2017 (Singing Dragon)

- *Compassionate Mindful Inquiry in Therapeutic Practice: A Practical Guide for Mindfulness Teachers, Yoga Teachers and Allied Health Professionals* by Karen Atkinson 2020 (Singing Dragon)

- Trauma-informed mindfulness. Meditation safety toolbox: www.brown.edu/research/labs/britton/meditation-safety-toolbox

References

Alwan, N.A. and Johnson, L. (2021) Defining long COVID: Going back to the start. *Med (NY)* 2(5):501–4.

Aylward, M. (2021) *Awake Where You Are: The Art of Embodied Awareness.* Wisdom.

BACME (British Association of Clinicians in ME) (2021) *An Introduction to Dysregulation in ME/CFS.*

Barhorst, E.E., Boruch, A.E., Cook, D.B. and Lindheimer, J.B. (2022) Pain-related post-exertional malaise in myalgic encephalomyelitis/chronic fatigue syndrome (ME/CFS) and fibromyalgia: A systematic review and three-level meta-analysis.' *Pain Medicine* 23(6):1144–57.

Bartley, T. (2011) *Mindfulness-based Cognitive Therapy for Cancer: Gently Turning Towards.* John Wiley & Sons.

Batchelor, S. (2017) The core concept of secular Buddhism: A fourfold-task. Accessed on 11 November 2022 at https://secularbuddhistnetwork.org/the-core-concept-of-secular-buddhism-a-fourfold-task

Bernardy, K., Klose, P., Welsch, P. and Häuser, W. (2018) Efficacy, acceptability and safety of cognitive behavioural therapies in fibromyalgia syndrome: A systematic review and meta-analysis of randomized controlled trials. *European Journal of Pain* 22(2):242–60.

Bishop, S.R. (2004) Mindfulness: A proposed operational definition. *Clinical Psychology: Science and Practice* 11(3):230–41.

Bisseling, E.M., Schellekens, M.P.J., Spinhoven, P., Compen, F.R., Speckens, A.E.M. and Lee, M.L. (2019) Therapeutic alliance – not therapist competence or group cohesion – contributes to reduction of psychological distress in group-based mindfulness-based cognitive therapy for cancer patients. *Clinical Psychology and Psychotherapy* 26(3):309–18.

Box, G.E.P. and Draper, N. (1987) *Empirical Model-building and Response Surfaces.* John Wiley & Sons.

Brach, T. (2013) *True Refuge: Finding Peace and Freedom in Your Own Awakened Heart.* Hay House.

Burch, V. and Penman, D. (2013) *Mindfulness for Health: A Practical Guide to Relieving Pain, Reducing Stress and Restoring Wellbeing.* Hachette.

Cheshire, A., Ridge, D., Clark, L.V. and White, P.D. (2020) Guided graded exercise self-help for chronic fatigue syndrome: Patient experiences and perceptions. *Disability and Rehabilitation* 42(3):368–77.

Cheshire, A., Ridge, D., Clark, L.V. and White, P.D. (2021) Sick of the sick role: Narratives of what 'recovery' means to people with CFS/ME. *Qualitative Health Research* 31(2):298–308.

Chew-Graham, C., Brooks, J., Wearden, A., Dowrick, C. and Peters, S. (2011) Factors influencing engagement of patients in a novel intervention for CFS/ME: A qualitative study. *Primary Health Care Research and Development* 12(2):112–22.

Chew-Graham, C., Dowrick, C., Wearden, A., Richardson, V. and Peters, S. (2010) Making the diagnosis of chronic fatigue syndrome/myalgic encephalitis in primary care: A qualitative study. *BMC Family Practice* 11(1):16.

Clark, J.E., Ng, W.F., Rushton, S., Watson, S. and Newton, J.L. (2019) Network structure underpinning (dys)homeostasis in chronic fatigue syndrome: Preliminary findings. *PLoS One* 14(3):e0213724.

Clauw, D.J. (2010) Perspectives on fatigue from the study of chronic fatigue syndrome and related conditions. *PM & R: The journal of injury, function, and rehabilitation* 2(5):414–30.

Coakley, G. and Knops, B. (2022) *Living with ME and Chronic Fatigue Syndrome.* Series: Penguin Life Expert Series #6 Imprint: Penguin Life.

Collin, S.M., Crawley, E., May, M.T., Sterne, J.A.C. and Hollingworth, W. (2011) The impact of CFS/ME on employment and productivity in the UK: A cross-sectional study based on the CFS/ME national outcomes database. *BMC Health Services Research* 11:217. doi:10.1186/1472-6963-11-217

Cox, D.L. (2000) *Occupational Therapy and Chronic Fatigue Syndrome.* Whurr.

Crane, C., Crane, R.S., Eames, C., Fennell, M.J.V. et al. (2014) The effects of amount of home meditation practice in mindfulness based cognitive therapy on hazard of relapse to depression in the Staying Well after Depression Trial. *Behaviour Research and Therapy* 63:17–24.

Crane, R.S. (2017a) Implementing mindfulness in the mainstream: Making the path by walking it. *Mindfulness* 8(3):585–94.

Crane, R.S. (2017b) *Mindfulness-based Cognitive Therapy: Distinctive Features.* Routledge.

Crane, R.S., Karunavira, and Griffith, G.M. (eds.) (2021) *Essential Resources for Mindfulness Teachers.* Routledge.

Davis, M.P. and Walsh, D. (2010) Mechanisms of fatigue. *Journal of Supportive Oncology* 8(4):164–74.

de Venter, M., Illegems, J., van Royen, R., Moorkens, G. et al. (2017) Differential effects of childhood trauma subtypes on fatigue and physical functioning in chronic fatigue syndrome. *Comprehensive Psychiatry* 78:76–82.

Durocher, E., Gibson, B.E. and Rappolt, S. (2014) Occupational justice: A conceptual review. *Journal of Occupational Science* 21(4):418–30.

Espeleta, H.C., Sharkey, C.M., Bakula, D.M., Gamwell, K.L. et al. (2020) Adverse childhood experiences and chronic medical conditions: Emotion dysregulation as a mediator of adjustment. *Journal of Clinical Psychology in Medical Settings* 27(3):572–81.

Feldman, C. and Kuyken, W. (2019) *Mindfulness: Ancient Wisdom Meets Modern Psychology.* Guilford.

Finsterer, J. and Mahjoub, S.Z. (2014) Fatigue in healthy and diseased individuals. *American Journal of Hospice and Palliative Medicine* 31(5):562–75.

Germer, C. (2009) *The Mindful Path to Self-Compassion: Freeing Yourself from Destructive Thoughts and Emotions.* Guilford.

Gilbert, P. (2010) *The Compassionate Mind: A New Approach to Life's Challenges.* Constable.

Gilbert, P. (2020) *Compassion: From Its Evolution to a Psychotherapy. Vol. 11: Frontiers in Psychology.* Frontiers Media.

Gilbert, P. and Choden (2013) *Mindful Compassion.* Hachette.

Griffith, G.M., Bartley, T. and Crane, R.S. (2019) The inside out group model: Teaching groups in mindfulness-based programs. *Mindfulness* 10(7):1315–27.

Hammond, C. (2019) *The Art of Rest: How to Find Respite in the Modern Age.* Canongate.

Hammond, C. and Lewis, G.T. (2016) The Rest Test: Preliminary Findings from a Large-Scale International Survey on Rest. In F. Callard, K. Staines and J. Wilkes (eds.) *The Restless Compendium,* pp.59–67. Palgrave Macmillan.

Hanson, R., Shapiro, S., Hutton-Thamm, E., Hagerty, M.R. and Sullivan, K.P. (2021) Learning to learn from positive experiences. *Journal of Positive Psychology* 1–12.

Hayes, S.C. and Smith, S. (2005) *Out of Your Mind and into Your Life: The New Acceptance and Commitment Therapy.* New Harbinger.

Heim, C., Nater, U.M., Maloney, E., Boneva, R., Jones, J.F. and Reeves, W.C. (2009) Childhood trauma and risk for chronic fatigue syndrome. *Archives of General Psychiatry* 66(1):72.

Hickie, I., Davenport, T., Vernon, S.D., Nisenbaum, R. et al. (2009) Are chronic fatigue and chronic fatigue syndrome valid clinical entities across countries and health-care settings? *Australian and New Zealand Journal of Psychiatry* 43(1):25–35.

Hocking, C., Townsend, E. and Mace, J. (2021) World Federation of Occupational Therapists position statement: Occupational Therapy and Human Rights (Revised 2019) – the backstory and future challenges. *World Federation of Occupational Therapists Bulletin,* 29 April, pp.1–7.

Jason, L.A., Evans, M., So, S., Scott, J. and Brown, A. (2015) Problems in defining post-exertional malaise. *Journal of Prevention and Intervention in the Community* 43(1):20–31.

Kabat-Zinn, J. (2013) *Full Catastrophe Living: How to Cope with Stress, Pain and Illness Using Mindfulness Meditation.* Hachette.

Kabat-Zinn, J. (2017) Defining mindfulness. Accessed on 11 November 2022 at www.mindful.org/jon-kabat-zinn-defining-mindfulness

Khanpour Ardestani, S., Karkhaneh, M., Stein, E., Punja, S. et al. (2021) Systematic review of mind-body interventions to treat myalgic encephalomyelitis/chronic fatigue syndrome. *Medicina (B. Aires)* 57(7):652.

Khoury, B., Lecomte, T., Fortin, G., Masse, M. et al. (2013) Mindfulness-based therapy: A comprehensive meta-analysis. *Clinical Psychology Review* 33(6):763–71.

Kielhofner, G. (ed.) (2002) *A Model of Human Occupation: Theory and Application.* Lippincott, Williams & Wilkins.

Kuyken, W., Hastings, R., Soulsby, J., Eames, C. et al. (2021) *Mindfulness-based Interventions: Teaching Assessment Criteria (MBI-TAC).* Available at https://mbitac.bangor.ac.uk/documents/MBITACmanual0517.pdf

Laird, K.T., Tanner-Smith, E.E., Russell, A.C., Hollon, S.D. and Walker, L.S. (2017) Comparative efficacy of psychological therapies for improving mental health and daily functioning in irritable bowel syndrome: A systematic review and meta-analysis. *Clinical Psychology Review* 51:142–52.

Larun, L. and Malterud, K. (2011) Finding the right balance of physical activity. *Patient Education and Counseling* 83(2):222–6.

Lee, D. and James, S. (2012) *The Compassionate Mind Approach to Recovering from Trauma: Using Compassion Focused Therapy.* Hachette.

Lewis, G. (2006) *Sunbathing in the Rain.* Harper Perennial.

Moghimi, N., di Napoli, M., Biller, J., Siegler, J.E. et al. (2021) The neurological manifestations of post-acute sequelae of SARS-CoV-2 infection. *Current Neurology and Neuroscience Reports* 21(9):44.

Morris, G., Maes, M., Berk, M. and Puri, B.K. (2019) Myalgic encephalomyelitis or chronic fatigue syndrome: How could the illness develop? *Metabolic Brain Disease* 34(2):385–415.

Nairn, R., Choden and Regan-Addis, H. (2019) *From Mindfulness to Insight: Meditations to Release Your Habitual Thinking and Activate Your Inherent Wisdom.* Shambhala.

NICE (2021a) *COVID 19 Rapid Guideline: Managing the Long-term Effects of COVID-19* [NG188]. Available at https://covid19-rapid-guideline-managing-the-longterm-effects-of-covid19-pdf-51035515742

NICE (2021b) *Chronic Pain (Primary and Secondary) in over 16s: Assessment of All Chronic Pain and Management of Chronic Primary Pain* [NG193]. Available at www.nice.org.uk/guidance/ng193

NICE (2021c). *Myalgic Encephalomyelitis (or Encephalopathy)/Chronic Fatigue Syndrome: Diagnosis and Management* [NG206]. Available at www.nice.org.uk/guidance/ng206

NICE (2022) *Depression in Adults: Treatment and Management* [NG222]. Available at www.nice.org.uk/guidance/ng222

Nijs, J., Meeus, M., van Oosterwijck, J., Ickmans, K. et al. (2012) In the mind or in the brain? Scientific evidence for central sensitisation in chronic fatigue syndrome. *European Journal of Clinical Investigation* 42(2):203–12.

Nin, A. (1975) *The Diary of Anaïs Nin, Vol 5: 1947–1955.* Houghton Mifflin Harcourt Publishing Company.

O'Dowd, B. and Griffith, G.M. (2022) 'I need to start listening to what my body is telling me': Does mindfulness-based cognitive therapy help people with chronic fatigue syndrome? *Human Arenas* 5(1):5–24.

Office for National Statistics (ONS) (2022) Prevalence of ongoing symptoms following coronavirus (COVID-19) infection in the UK. Statistical Bulletin. Accessed on 9 November 2022 at www.ons.gov.uk/peoplepopulationandcommunity/healthandsocialcare/conditionsanddiseases/bulletins/prevalenceofongoingsymptomsfollowingcoronaviruscovid19infectionintheuk/3november2022#cite-this-statistical-bulletin

Parkinson, S., Forsyth, K. and Kielhofner, G. (2004) *A User's Manual for the Model of Human Occupation Screening Tool (MOHOST).* University of Illinois at Chicago.

Pilkington, K., Ridge, D.T., Igwesi-Chidobe, C.N., Chew-Graham, C.A. et al. (2020) A relational analysis of an invisible illness: A meta-ethnography of people with chronic fatigue syndrome/myalgic encephalomyelitis (CFS/ME) and their support needs. *Social Science and Medicine* 265:113369. doi:10.1016/j.socscimed.2020.113369

Pinker, S. (2015) *The Sense of Style: The Thinking Person's Guide to Writing in the 21st Century.* Penguin.

Pizga, A., Kordoutis, P., Tsikrika, S., Vasileiadis, I., Nanas, S. and Karatzanos, E. (2021) Effects of cognitive behavioral therapy on depression, anxiety, sleep and quality of life for patients with heart failure and coronary heart disease: A systematic review of clinical trials 2010–2020. *Health and Research Journal* 7(3):123.

Pole, N. (2017) *Words that Touch: How to Ask Questions Your Body Can Answer – 12 Essential 'Clean Questions' for Mind/Body Therapists.* Singing Dragon.

Pollak, S.M., Pedulla, T. and Siegel, R.D. (2014) *Sitting Together: Essential Skills for Mindfulness-based Psychotherapy.* Guilford.

Popper, K. (2005) *The Logic of Scientific Discovery.* Routledge.

Porges, S.W. (2007) The polyvagal perspective. *Biological Psychology* 74(2):116–43.

Ray, R. (2016) *The Awakening Body: Somatic Meditation for Discovering Our Deepest Life.* Shambhala.

Reeves, W.C., Jones, J.F., Maloney, E., Heim, C. et al. (2007) Prevalence of chronic fatigue syndrome in metropolitan, urban, and rural Georgia. *Population Health Metrics* 5(1):5.

Ribeiro, L., Atchley, R.M. and Oken, B.S. (2018) Adherence to practice of mindfulness in novice meditators: Practices chosen, amount of time practiced, and long-term effects following a mindfulness-based intervention. *Mindfulness* 9(2):401–11.

Rimes, K.A. and Wingrove, J. (2013) Mindfulness-based cognitive therapy for people with chronic fatigue syndrome still experiencing excessive fatigue after cognitive behaviour therapy: A pilot randomized study. *Clinical Psychology and Psychotherapy* 20(2):107–17.

Rivas-Vazquez, R.A., Rey, G., Quintana, A. and Rivas-Vazquez, A.A. (2022) Assessment and management of long COVID. *Journal of Health Service Psychology* 48(1):21–30.

Routen, A., O'Mahoney, L., Ayoubkhani, D., Banerjee, A. et al. (2022) Understanding and tracking the impact of long COVID in the United Kingdom. *Nature Medicine* 28(1):11–15.

Royal College of Physicians (2022) *The Diagnosis of Fibromyalgia Syndrome: UK Clinical Guidelines.* Available at www.rcp.ac.uk/guidelines-policy/diagnosis-fibromyalgia-syndrome

Rumi, J (1995) *The Essential Rumi: A Poetry Anthology* (C. Barks, Trans.). Harper Collins.

Rycroft-Malone, J., Gradinger, F., Griffiths, H.O., Crane, R. et al. (2017) Accessibility and implementation in the UK NHS services of an effective depression relapse prevention programme: Learning from mindfulness-based cognitive therapy through a mixed-methods study. *Health Services and Delivery Research* 5(14):1–190.

Santorelli, S.F., Meleo-Meyer, F., Koerbel, L. and Kabat-Zinn, J. (2017) *Mindfulness-based Stress Reduction (MBSR) Authorized Curriculum Guide.* Center for Mindfulness in Medicine, Healthcare, and Society, University of Massachusetts Medical School.

Segal, Z., Williams, M. and Teasdale, J. (2013) *Mindfulness-based Cognitive Therapy for Depression.* Guilford.

Shan, Z.Y., Barnden, L.R., Kwiatek, R.A., Bhuta, S., Hermens, D.F. and Lagopoulos, J. (2020) Neuroimaging characteristics of myalgic encephalomyelitis/chronic fatigue syndrome (ME/CFS): A systematic review. *Journal of Translational Medicine* 18(1):335. doi:10.1186/s12967-020-02506-6

Shapiro, S.L., Carlson, L.E., Astin, J.A. and Freedman, B. (2006) Mechanisms of mindfulness. *Journal of Clinical Psychology* 62(3):373–86.

Sharpe, M. and Greco, M. (2019) Chronic fatigue syndrome and an illness-focused approach to care: Controversy, morality and paradox. *Medical Humanities* 45(2):183–7.

Shepherd, C. and Chaudhuri, A. (2020) *ME/CFS/PVFs: An Exploration of Key Clinical Issues* (12th edn). ME Association.

Siegel, D. (1999) *The Developing Mind.* Guilford.

Strohmaier, S., Jones, F.W. and Cane, J.E. (2021) Effects of length of mindfulness practice on mindfulness, depression, anxiety, and stress: A randomized controlled experiment. *Mindfulness* 12(1):198–214.

Stussman, B., Williams, A., Snow, J., Gavin, A. et al. (2020) Characterization of post-exertional malaise in patients with myalgic encephalomyelitis/chronic fatigue syndrome. *Frontiers in Neurology* 11:1025. doi:10.3389/fneur.2020.01025

Surawy, C., Hackmann, A., Hawton, K. and Sharpe, M. (1995) Chronic fatigue syndrome: A cognitive approach. *Behaviour Research and Therapy* 33(5):535–44.

Surawy, C., Roberts, J. and Silver, A. (2005) The effect of mindfulness training on mood and measures of fatigue, activity, and quality of life in patients with chronic fatigue syndrome on a hospital waiting list: A series of exploratory studies. *Behavioural and Cognitive Psychotherapy* 33(1):103–9.

Swain, M.G. (2000) Fatigue in chronic disease. *Clinical Science* 99(1):1–8.

Taylor, R.R., Kielhofner, G.W., Abelenda, J., Colantuono, K. et al. (2003) An approach to persons with chronic fatigue syndrome based on the model of human occupation: Part one, Impact on occupational performance and participation. *Occupational Therapy in Health Care* 17(2):47–61.

Teodoro, T., Edwards, M.J. and Isaacs, J.D. (2018) A unifying theory for cognitive abnormalities in functional neurological disorders, fibromyalgia and chronic fatigue syndrome: Systematic review. *Journal of Neurology, Neurosurgery and Psychiatry* 89(12):1308–19.

Treleaven, D.A. (2018) *Trauma-sensitive Mindfulness: Practices for Safe and Transformative Healing.* W.W. Norton & Co.

Twomey, R., Yeung, S.T., Wrightson, J.G., Millet, G.Y. and Culos-Reed, S.N. (2020) Post-exertional malaise in people with chronic cancer-related fatigue. *Journal of Pain and Symptom Management* 60(2):407–16.

UK Network of Mindfulness Teacher Training Organisations (2015) *Good Practice Guidance for Teachers (April 2015).* Available from https://bamba.org.uk/wp-content/uploads/2019/06/UK-MB-teacher-GPG-2015-final-2.pdf

Unity Health (n.d.) *Mindfulness and the Window of Tolerance.* Accessed on 1 November 2022 at https://unityhealth.to/wp-content/uploads/2021/07/mast-session1.pdf?msclkid=3d44befbba3d11ec94ae9bad1aef61f

van Dam, N.T., van Vugt, M.K., Vago, D.R., Schmalzl, L. et al. (2018) Mind the hype: A critical evaluation and prescriptive agenda for research on mindfulness and meditation. *Perspectives on Psychological Science* 13(1):36–61.

van der Kolk, B. (2014) *The Body Keeps the Score: Mind, Brain and Body in the Transformation of Trauma.* Penguin.

Varela, F.J., Thompson, E. and Rosch, E. (2017) *The Embodied Mind: Cognitive Science and Human Experience.* MIT Press.

Weir, W. and Speight, N. (2021) ME/CFS: Past, present and future. *Healthcare* 9(8):984.

Wellings, N. (2016) *Why Can't I Meditate? How to Get Your Mindfulness Practice on Track.* TarcherPerigee.

Wessely, S., Chalder, T., Hirsch, S., Wallace, P. and Wright, D. (1997) The prevalence and morbidity of chronic fatigue and chronic fatigue syndrome: A prospective primary care study. *American Journal of Public Health* 87(9):1449–55.

Whyte, D. (2019) *Consolations: The Solace, Nourishment and Underlying Meaning of Everyday Words.* Canongate.

Williams, J.M.G., Baer, R., Batchelor, M., Crane, R.S. et al. (2022) What next after MBSR/MBCT? An open trial of an 8-week follow-on program exploring mindfulness of feeling tone (*vedanā*). *Mindfulness* 13(8):1931–44.

Williams, J.M.G., Teasdale, J.D., Segal, Z. and Kabat-Zinn, J. (2007) *The Mindful Way Through Depression: Freeing Yourself from Chronic Unhappiness.* Guilford.

Williams, M. and Penman, D. (2011) *A Practical Guide to Finding Peace in a Frantic World.* Piatkus.

Wurz, A., Culos-Reed, S.N., Franklin, K., DeMars, J. et al. (2022) 'I feel like my body is broken': Exploring the experiences of people living with long COVID. *Quality of Life Research* 31(12):3339–54.

Yorkston, K.M., Johnson, K., Boesflug, E., Skala, J. and Amtmann, D. (2010) Communicating about the experience of pain and fatigue in disability. *Quality of Life Research* 19(2):243–51.

Index

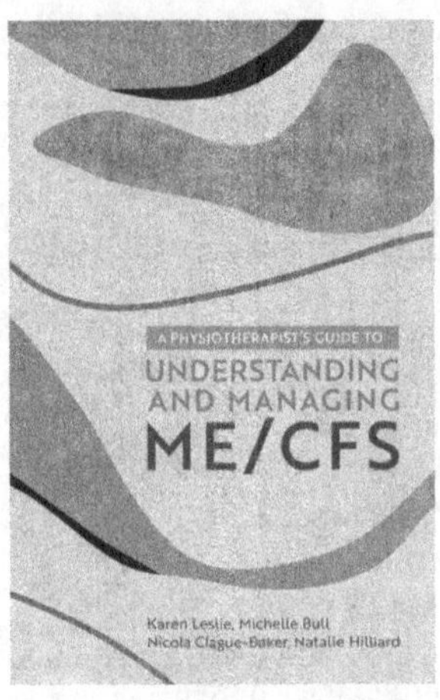

A Physiotherapist's Guide to Understanding and Managing ME/CFS

Karen Leslie, Michelle Bull, Nicola Clague-Baker, Natalie Hilliard

£26.99 | $35.00 | PB | 320PP |
ISBN 978 1 83997 143 3 |
eISBN 978 1 83997 144 0

Myalgic encephalomyelitis (ME), also known as chronic fatigue syndrome (CFS), is a deeply complex and multi-system condition which has historically suffered from a ack of awareness within physiotherapy education and practice. Similarities in presentation between this condition and Long Covid make this comprehensive and evidence-based guide for physiotherapists even more timely and important.

This guide includes an in-depth explanation and history of ME/CFS, while also describing symptoms, varying degrees of severity and how to manage ME/CFS in children. It also provides detailed management advice and discussion on how the information can directly inform physiotherapy practice, supplemented with patient case studies.

Karen Leslie is a Chartered Physiotherapist specializing in neurological rehabilitation. She works in private practice and has a background in journalism and communications.

Dr Michelle Bull qualified as a Chartered Physiotherapist over 30 years ago and has worked in clinical and non-clinical roles with an emphasis on cardiac rehabilitation, cancer rehabilitation, physical activity promotion and Long Covid.

Dr Nicola Clague-Baker is a Chartered Physiotherapist with over 30 years' experience. She currently teaches neurological physiotherapy at the University of Liverpool and leads research on ME/CFS and Long Covid.

Natalie Hilliard works clinically as a Chartered Physiotherapist in private practice, covering musculoskeletal and neurological conditions and specializing in the management of ME/CFS and Long Covid.

The authors have clinical and personal experience of ME/CFS and are Co-Founders of Physios for ME, an organization aiming to address the issues around physiotherapy provision for people with ME/CFS. They are based in England.

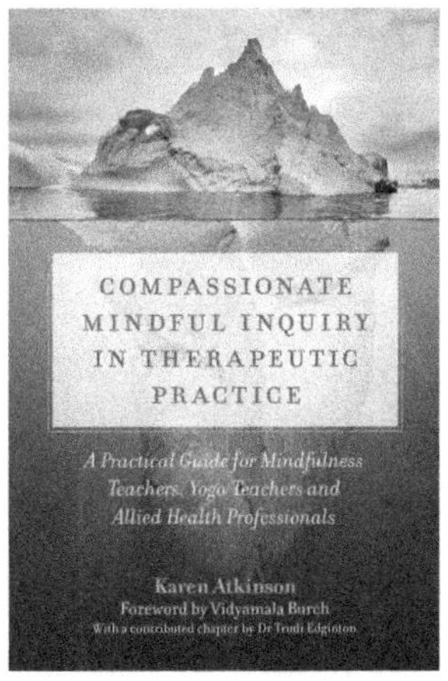

Compassionate Mindful Inquiry in Therapeutic Practice

A Practical Guide for Mindfulness Teachers, Yoga Teachers and Allied Health Professionals

Karen Atkinson

Foreword by Vidyamala Burch

£17.99 | $24.95 | PB | 192PP |
ISBN 978 1 78775 175 0 |
eISBN 978 1 78775 176 7

Practical and informative, this hands-on manual clearly depicts the relationship between mindfulness and compassion, demonstrating how one supports the other. This book offers a fresh perspective on mindfulness that resonates with a human approach and helps practitioners to validate their work by giving a sense of grounding and direction, and providing a safe, appropriate and transformative process in which to conduct inquiry.

Including chapters on the meaning of Compassionate Mindful Inquiry and the Model of Inquiry, Atkinson facilitates transformational change and offers guidance for those incorporating mindfulness teaching into their own professional practice, whilst Dr Trudi Edginton explains the neuroscience behind these processes.

Karen Atkinson is the Senior Partner and Co-Founder of MindfulnessUK. She is also on the executive committee for the British Association of Mindfulness-Based Approaches, which upholds standards and builds integrity in the mindfulness field.

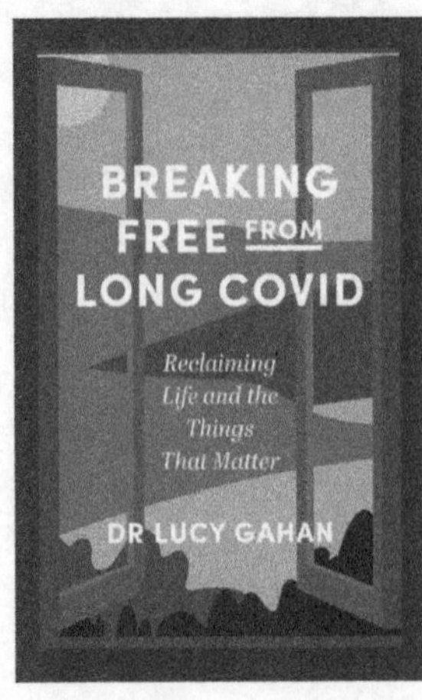

Breaking Free from Long Covid

Reclaiming Life and the Things That Matter

Dr Lucy Gahan

£12.99 | $18.95 | PB | 192PP |
ISBN 978 1 83997 350 5 |
eISBN 978 1 83997 351 2

Making visible the real effects of Long Covid on people and their lives, this guide explores the issues of living with the condition.

Rooted in the author's own experience of having Long Covid since April 2020, the book offers ideas from narrative therapy as a lens through which to address the emotional impact of the condition, and shares practical strategies for managing symptoms and regaining quality of life. Acknowledging that recovery is unpredictable, it sheds light on the often invisible challenges faced by people living with chronic conditions, such as managing pacing and rest in a world that values productivity, the impact of illness on relationships, coping in the context of a pandemic and negotiating day-to-day life when you are living between illness and wellness.

Dr Lucy Gahan is a clinical psychologist who, after a long period of absence from work due to Long Covid, is now part of an NHS Long Covid team. With previous roles as a psychologist in palliative care, as a physiotherapy assistant and in the fitness industry, her passions lie in working with the mind and body. She has had Long Covid since April 2020. She regularly fails to pace herself.